| DR. MEHBOOB H. KUKASWADIA
Family Doctor
No. 2 Maryborough Court,
Maryborough Hill,
Douglas, Cork.
.Tel. 021-361504

PRESENTED TO:

DR M. AKHTAR
CODE 1024
PMC PHYSICIAN

Third Edition

THE
BEECHAM MANUAL
FOR
FAMILY PRACTICE

Third Edition

THE BEECHAM MANUAL FOR FAMILY PRACTICE

Edited by Dr John Fry

in association with

Dr E. C. Gambrill
Dr A. J. Moulds
Dr Gillian Strube

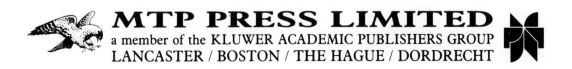

MTP PRESS LIMITED
a member of the KLUWER ACADEMIC PUBLISHERS GROUP
LANCASTER / BOSTON / THE HAGUE / DORDRECHT

This book was originally issued in 3 volumes under the title *A Manual for General Practice,* by Beecham Research Laboratories, Beecham House, Great West Road, Brentford, Middlesex TW8 9BD.

Published in the UK and Europe by
MTP Press Limited
Falcon House
Lancaster, England.

British Library Cataloguing in Publication Data

The Beecham manual for family practice.
   1. Family medicine
   I. Fry, John, *1922–*
   362.1'72   R729.5.G4

ISBN 0-85200-911-9

Published in the USA by
MTP Press
A division of Kluwer Boston Inc.
190 Old Derby Street
Hingham, MA 02043, USA.

Library of Congress Cataloguing in Publication Data

Main entry under title:

The Beecham manual for family practice.

   Includes index.
   1. Family medicine.   I. Fry, John.
[DNLM: 1. Family Practice—handbooks. WB 39 B414]
RC46.B43   1985   616   85-11485
ISBN 0-85200-911-9

Typeset by UPS Blackburn Ltd., Northgate, Blackburn BB2 1AB and Printed and bound in Great Britain by Butler and Tanner Limited, Frome and London

Contents

Foreword

This third edition of the *Beecham Manual* has its origins in a manual produced by Selwyn Carson for his general practice in Christchurch, New Zealand. He produced loose-leaf sets of instructions for his practice team and colleagues. Beecham Research Laboratories of New Zealand did a great service for the medical profession by publishing and distributing Dr Carson's manual there.

The British version of the *Beecham Manual* had different objectives. The vocational training programme needed basic resources and the British *Manual* was created as an easy to read reference book on common problems and methods in general practice.

The first and second editions met with enthusiastic approval from principals, trainers and trainees. This third edition follows the same general format but has been completely revised and updated and includes many new additions. The five sections are:

- ○ planned care of definable population and other groups
- ○ principles of teaching and learning
- ○ emergencies and their management
- ○ psychiatry
- ○ clinical care of common conditions

We have kept to simple, clear and brief presentations of our conjoint views based on our experiences in our own practices.

We dedicate this third edition to our colleagues involved in caring, learning and teaching. They may not agree with us completely but we hope that we will make them consider our suggestions and use them for thought, debate and discussion. We hope also that it will be used as a work book for the whole practice team.

We thank Beecham Research Laboratories (BRL) for their continuing support and for the complete independence given to us.

To Bill Burns of BRL go our special thanks for encouraging and organising us and to David Bloomer of MTP for turning our manuscripts into finished products.

John Fry
June 1985

Section A

PLANNED CARE

A1 Family Planning

Discuss with the individual patient the advantages and disadvantages of all the methods. Keep in mind individual needs, wishes and religious beliefs.

In Great Britain

○ 2.5 million women are registered with their GPs for contraception – 80–90 per GP.
○ 97% of GPs provide contraceptive services.
○ 20% of GPs fit IUCDs.
○ Up to 10% of married couples are involuntarily infertile.
○ 1.66 is the average number of children per family.
○ The population is decreasing slightly.
○ 1 in 10 pregnancies end in a natural abortion – 2–3 per GP.
○ 120000 induced abortions per annum – 4–5 per GP.
○ Premaritally conceived births by girls under 20 dropped by 50% in the past decade.
○ Less than 1% of women who use NHS family planning clinics are under the age of 16.

Current contraceptive usage by sexually active women:

Method	'General' women (831) %	New mothers (200) %
Oral contraception	36	52
IUCD	6	8
Diaphragm [1]	1	1
Sheath	15	12
Safe period	1	2
Chemicals alone	1	0
Withdrawal	3	1
None	13	10
Vasectomy [2]	10	4
Female sterilization[3]	8	7

Adapted from Allen, 1981

[1] Many more women have tried the diaphragm than continue using it
[2] Vasectomy is increasing in popularity. 35% of 30–35-year-old women come from marriages with vasectomy as the method of contraception
[3] Around 100000 female sterilizations are performed each year

Pregnancy failure
rates for different
methods of
contraception

Total pregnancy rate (method and patient failure) per 100 woman-years.

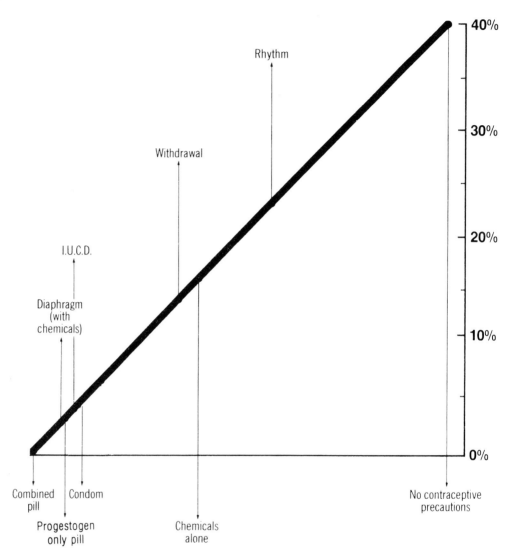

○ The overall failure rate of vasectomy and sterilization is less than 0.5 per 100 patients.
○ Postcoital contraceptive methods have a failure rate of about 1 per 100 occasions on which the method is used.

Usage of family planning services by sexually active women:

	'General' women (922) %	New mothers (200) %
Ever used both GP/FP clinic	26	36
Only ever used GP	38	52
Only ever used FP clinic [1]	12	7
Total ever usage FP services	76	95

Adapted from Allen, 1981

[1] Most women use general practice as their primary source of family planning advice

Degree of satisfaction among users of family planning services:

	GP services (527) %	FP clinics (358) %
Very satisfied	50	53
Satisfied	22	22
Quite satisfied	15	15
Not very satisfied	7[1]	5
Not satisfied	3[1]	4
Don't know	3	1

Adapted from Allen, 1981

[1] There are 3 main areas where patients find GP family planning services less than satisfactory:

(1) delays in obtaining appointments
(2) doctors perceived as being too busy to spend adequate time on the subject
(3) obtrusive and aggressive questioning by receptionists and other members of the staff

The Combined Pill

Various oestrogen and progestogen combination pills are taken by 3 million women in Great Britain and, with sterilization, form by far the most effective means of contraception known. The pill is a source of great public interest and debate. Although serious complications are rare the doctor must be well informed about possible adverse effects and organize regular super-vision.

Starting a Patient on the Pill

The oral contraceptive most suited to a particular woman is often found by trial and error. The aim should always be to use the lowest possible dose of both hormones that will achieve good cycle control. Family Planning Association approved pills are Brevinor, Ovysmen, Neocon 1/35, Norimin, Microgynon 30, Ovranette, Marvelon, Binovum, Trinovum, Logynon and Trinordiol.

Patients changing from one preparation to another containing a reduced level of either or both hormones should be advised to take additional precautions for the first 14 days.

The pill should be stopped at least 1 month prior to any major surgical operation or if there is likely to be prolonged immobility for any reason.

Advice to the patient
(when starting or restarting the pill)

1. Explain what the 'pill' is and how it works.

2. Counting the first day of your period as day 1 then take the first pill on day 5 whether your period has finished or not. Use additional precautions for the first 14 days.
   or Start on day 1 and use no other precautions.

   N.B. In the first cycle all triphasic and biphasic pills are started on the first day.

3. Take the pill at the same time each day.

4. When the packet is finished stop for 7 days, during which time you will have your period, then start your next course.

5. If you forget to take a pill, take one as soon as you remember. If the gap is more than 12 hours then do not take the pills you have forgotten but take the next one at the usual time and use additional precautions for the rest of that month.

6. If you have vomiting or diarrhoea lasting more than a few hours then continue the course but use additional precautions for the rest of it.

7. Mention – lightening of periods
   – break through bleeding
   – possible side effects

Notes

○ After a miscarriage or abortion the pill can be started after 5 days with an additional form of contraception used for the first 14 days.

○ After childbirth, waiting for the first period before starting the pill allows the endocrine system to recover from the hormonal changes of pregnancy. However, if effective contraception is needed, the pill can be started 5 days after parturition, provided the woman is recovered and active. If breast feeding, then the progestogen only pill or sheath are preferable until the baby is off the breast.

○ Women on constant dose combined pills who wish to miss a period can be advised to take two or more packets consecutively without any pill-free days.

○ If a period is missed by a woman taking the pill then pregnancy should be excluded before a new course of pills is started.

○ Minor side effects like nausea, bloating, mild break through bleeding will usually disappear within the first 3 months.

○ Women stopping the pill to try to become pregnant should be advised to use some other form of contraception until they have had one true period.

○ 'Coming off' the pill at intervals does not enhance future fertility and may result in an unplanned pregnancy.

Oral contraceptives available in the UK

	Low dose preparations	
	Oestrogen	*Progestogen*
Loestrin 20	0.020 mg ethinyloestradiol	1.00 mg norethisterone acetate
Loestrin 30	0.030 mg ethinyloestradiol	1.50 mg norethisterone acetate
Marvelon*	0.030 mg ethinyloestradiol	0.15 desogestrel
Microgynon 30*/Ovranette*	0.030 mg ethinyloestradiol	0.15 mg levonorgestrel
Ovysmen*/Brevinor*	0.035 mg ethinyloestradiol	0.50 mg norethisterone[1]
Neocon 1/35*/Norimin*	0.035 mg ethinyloestradiol	1.00 mg norethisterone

Phasic preparations

I. *Constant dose of oestrogen with 'phased' norethisterone:*

Trinovum*	0.035 mg ethinyloestradiol	0.05/0.075/1.00 mg norethisterone
Bi-novum*	0.035 mg ethinyloestradiol	0.05/1.00 mg norethisterone

II. *Phased oestrogen with 'phased' levonorgestrel:*

Trinordiol*/Logynon*	0.030/0.04/0.03 mg ethinyl-oestradiol	0.05/0.075/0.125 mg levonorgestrel

Medium dose preparations

Eugynon 30/Ovran30	0.030 mg ethinyloestradiol	0.25 mg levonorgestrel
Conova 30	0.030 mg ethinyloestradiol	2.00 mg ethynodiol diacetate
Orthonovin 1/50/Norinyl 1	0.05 mg mestranol	1.00 mg norethisterone
Ovulen 50	0.05 mg ethinyloestradiol	1.00 mg ethynodiol diacetate
Orlest 21/Minovlar (ED)	0.05 mg ethinyloestradiol	1.00 mg norethisterone acetate
Norlestrin	0.05 mg ethinyloestradiol	2.50 mg norethisterone acetate
Gynovlar 21	0.05 mg ethinyloestradiol	3.00 mg norethisterone acetate
Anovlar 21	0.05 mg ethinyloestradiol	4.00 mg norethisterone acetate
Ovran	0.05 mg ethinyloestradiol	0.25 mg levonorgestrel
Eugynon 50	0.05 mg ethinyloestradiol	0.50 mg norgestrel
Minilyn	0.05 mg ethinyloestradiol	2.50 mg lynoestrenol

* Family Planning Association approved pills
[1] Norethisterone is the least powerful progestogen

History and examination

FAMILY PLANNING CARD	DOCTOR	
Name	Date of Birth	Address

PAST HISTORY/RISK FACTORS

PILL over 35 smoker overweight	hyperlipidaemia hypertension diabetes	jaundice migraine CVS disease
COIL/MINI PILL	ectopic pregnancy pelvic inflammation abdominal operations	OTHERS

GYNAE ASSESSMENT

PARA	CYCLE	PELVIC EXAM

SCREENING

RUBELLA	SMEAR	BREAST LEAFLET/EXAM

DATE	BP	NOTES	1001 1002

This record card, used by Laindon Health Centre, Basildon, Essex, sums up the main areas of history and examination. LMP and any regular medication would also be included.

A pelvic examination is desirable to exclude pregnancy or pelvic pathology. However, in the absence of symptoms suggesting a medical need for such an examination, it need not be insisted on. In some cases it may put women off attending for contraceptive care.

Routine follow-up	1.	Blood pressure – record 6 monthly.

Routine follow-up

1. Blood pressure – record 6 monthly.

2. Weight – record initial baseline only.

3. Pelvic examination – at some stage before or in the first year of pill taking. Otherwise only if there is a clinical indication.

4. Smear test – after been sexually active for 1–2 years then every 5 years thereafter.

5. Breast examination – may be carried out to exclude malignancy. Teaching self-examination and providing a suitable leaflet, particularly to the over-30s, may be worth considering.

Possible complications

A. **Deep vein thrombosis**
4 times greater than in a non-user. Not related to duration of use, oestrogen dose or progestogen content, or to presence of varicose veins.

B. **Superficial thrombosis**
2.5 times greater than in a non-user. Not related to duration of use but significantly related to both oestrogen dose and progestogen content. Also related to presence and severity of varicose veins.

C. **Circulatory diseases**
Deaths from a wide range of vascular conditions of 1 per 5000 ever users per year. Related to duration of use, age and cigarette smoking; also obesity and diseases predisposing to vascular complications, e.g. diabetes.

D. **Hypertension**
Up to 5% of users will develop this after 5 years. In most cases is reversible. Do not assume that this is caused by the pill.

E. **Cancer**
Prolonged pill use appears to be associated with an increased risk of carcinoma of the cervix. Regular cytological screening can reduce this risk. Extremely rarely the pill is also associated with the development of primary hepatocellular carcinoma.

At present it is not possible to say whether or not prolonged use of the pill by young women leads to a higher incidence of cancer of the breast.

Pill use decreases the incidence of cancer of the ovary and cancer of the body of the uterus.

F. **Fertility**
Pill use does not impair subsequent fertility.

G. **Pregnancy**
The risks of taking the pill are generally less than those of a pregnancy. The risk of the fetus being harmed in a 'pill pregnancy' is 1 in 1000; this should be compared with the background risk in any pregnancy of 20 in 1000 for important birth defects.

To minimize the risk of serious complications developing, the pill containing the lowest effective dose of both hormones, consistent with good cycle control, should be used.

Possible side effects and remedial action

First ever migraine attack or exacerbation of pre-existing migraine
Persistent severe headaches
Acute visual disturbances
Pregnancy
Jaundice
Moderate or severe hypertension
First signs of thrombophlebitis or thromboembolism

Action: Stop the pill

Bloating
Breast discomfort
Non-migrainous headaches
Mild hypertension
Recurrent migraine
Nausea and vomiting
Premenstrual tension
Vaginal (mucoid) discharge
Cyclical weight gain

Action: Reduce oestrogen dose

Acne
Breast discomfort
Depression (rule out psychogenic cause)
Dry vagina
Hirsutism
Loss of libido (rule out psychogenic cause)
Missed withdrawal bleeding
Steady weight gain (check dietary factors)

Action: Reduce progestogen dose

Heavy bleeding
Break through bleeding
Missed withdrawal bleeding (patient on low dose pill)

Action: Increase progestogen dose

Break through bleeding on lower dose pills (if increased
progestogen has not helped)

Action: Increase oestrogen dose

Contraindications

Absolute

1. Cardiovascular: History of thromboembolism
   Any existing vascular abnormality, e.g.
   any cause of pulmonary hypertension
   Severe hypertension
   Post splenectomy

2. Impaired liver function: Biliary cirrhosis
   Jaundice
   Recent or severe liver disease
   Impaired hepatic excretion
   History of idiopathic jaundice of pregnancy
   Dubin–Johnson or rotor syndrome

3. Carcinoma of the breast and genital tract

4. Major haemoglobinopathy

5. Porphyria

6. Deterioration of otosclerosis in pregnancy

Relative

In these cases oral contraceptives represent a lesser risk than pregnancy should no other method be acceptable or sufficiently effective. Further investigations or specialist opinion may be required before a decision to prescribe is taken. Careful follow-up is required.

1. Hypertension
2. Women over the age of 35 particularly if they are smokers or over-weight or a hypertensive or a diabetic or hyperlipidaemic or if they have a family history of CHD
3. Obesity
4. Severe migraine
5. Cervical dysplasia
6. Diabetes
7. Depression or other severe mood disorder
8. Familial hyperlipidaemia
9. Oligomenorrhoea or secondary amenorrhoea
10. Pre-existing neuro-ophthalmic disorders, eg MS
11. Otosclerosis
12. Lactation
13. Liver disorder

Notes

○ The pill should not be prescribed following a hydatidiform mole until human chorionic gonadotrophin is undetectable in the serum. Once the level is undetectable the pill is likely to be the method of choice.

○ Asthma may be exacerbated by concomitant oral contraceptive usage.

○ Women with epilepsy on anticonvulsant drugs like phenobarbitone, phenytoin, carbamazepine, should be prescribed a higher dose (0.05mg ethinyloestradiol) pill.

Drug interactions

Reduced contraceptive action

Concomitant administration of these drugs may reduce contraceptive efficacy. Break through bleeding or spotting following the taking of the drugs should be regarded as a warning sign.

Phenytoin	Rifampicin
Phenobarbitone	Griseofulvin
Primidone	Spironolactone
Ethosuximide	Chlordiazepoxide
Carbamazepine	Chlorpromazine
Dihydroergotamine	Diazepam
Aminocaproic acid	Meprobamate
Glutethamide	Antihistamines

N.B. Antibiotics may also cause contraceptive failure in women taking the pill. The interaction appears to be rare (the Committee on Safety of Medicines have had 38 reports) and it is not possible to predict which women are at risk. Cotrimoxazole may actually make the pill more effective.

Interference with the effect of other drugs

Hypoglycaemics	(∇)
Systemic corticosteroids	(Δ or ∇)
Anticoagulants	(∇)
Antidepressants	(∇)
Diuretics	(∇)

The Morning-after Pill

Uses

As an occasional emergency measure – e.g. after an accident with a sheath; after first time or 'unexpected' unprotected intercourse; after rape.

Method

○ Risk of conception after midcycle exposure is only 10–30% and falls to less than 10% at other times. Significant risk is from days 7 to 17 of a 28-day cycle.

○ Effective (failure rate about 1–2%) until 72 hours after the earliest unprotected intercourse in that cycle.

○ Use two tablets of Eugynon 50 or Ovran stat and in 12 hours. If either dose is vomited patient must take two additional tablets or, if a high pregnancy risk case, consider fitting an IUCD.

Advice to patient

1. Take two tablets now and another two in 12 hours time. If either dose is vomited within 3 hours then take a further two tablets or contact the surgery for advice.

2. Abstain from intercourse or use the sheath until the next menstrual period.

3. Failure of this method is possible. You must attend for follow-up in about 3 weeks (time about 1 week after the expected onset of the next period).

4. Your next period may come early.

5. If your next period does not come or if it is unexpectedly light then bring an early morning urine sample with you.

Follow-up

Follow-up visit is essential. Exclude ectopic or established pregnancy and discuss future family planning. Keep careful records.

The Progestogen only Pill

Uses

Alternative to the combined pill for women in whom oestrogens are contraindicated, e.g. diabetes, history of thromboembolism, hypertension with the combined pill, and who are prepared to accept the slightly increased risk of pregnancy.

Women over the age of 40 as their fertility is less and age dependent complications of oestrogen are increasing.

During lactation.

Types available

Name	Progestogen
Micronor/Noriday	0.35 mg norethisterone
Femulen	0.5 mg ethynodiol diacetate
Neogest	0.075 mg norgestrel
Microval/Norgeston	0.3 mg levonorgestrel

Starting

If no previous oral contraception then same history and examination as for the combined pill.

If changing over from the combined pill then must take additional precautions until have completed first 14 days on the progestogen only pill.

Contraindications

Levonorgestrel is the only progestogen that has no oestrogenic activity.

Absolute – history of ectopic pregnancy
undiagnosed menstrual irregularity
malignant disease of the breast

Relative – malabsorption syndrome
severe liver disorders with persistent biochemical change
after cone biopsy of the cervix

Advice to patient

1. Take the pill on the first day of your next period.

2. Take one pill every day thereafter without a break, whether menstruation occurs or not.

3. Take at any regular time you like except at bedtime if that is the time you most commonly have intercourse. (For most women the best time is between 6 and 7 p.m.)

4. Take extra contraceptive precautions – use the sheath – for 14 days:

   (a) after you first start taking the pill

   (b) if the pill is taken more than 3 hours late

   (c) if a pill is forgotten – take it when you realize your mistake then take the usual pill for that day at the usual time

   (d) if you have an attack of diarrhoea – take the pill as usual but take extra precautions for 14 days after the diarrhoea has stopped

   (e) if vomiting occurs within 2 hours of pill taking then take another – if it is also vomited then take the pill as usual but take extra precautions for 14 days after the vomiting has stopped

5.   Mention – irregularity of periods especially in the first few months.
     – return if two consecutive periods are missed.

Follow-up   As for the combined pill.

**Possible side   Much less than for the combined pill apart from
effects**   ○ cycle irregularity
                       ○ intermenstrual bleeding

Injectable Progestogen

Depo-Provera (medroxyprogesterone acetate) has recently been licensed for long term use. The CSM recommend that it should not be regarded as a first choice contraceptive agent. The licensing panel felt it 'would be a useful method of contraception for women for whom other contraceptives are contraindicated, cause side effects or are otherwise unsuitable and who are seeking long term contraception, provided they understand and accept the risks of side effects and uncertain delay in return to fertility.'

The Sheath

Uses

Couples where the male wishes to take responsibility for contraception.

Temporary protection while waiting to use other methods or while waiting for other methods to become effective.

For casual sex as is only method to give some protection against venereal disease.

Advice to patient

1. No medical prescription or supervision required.

2. Sheath only put on when penis is erect, before any contact with vulva.

3. The closed end of the sheath should be squeezed between thumb and forefinger to expel surplus air, then gently unrolled fully and evenly over the entire length of the penis. Some women do this for their partner as part of lovemaking.

4. After ejaculation the sheath should be held close to the penis so that it remains in place until the penis has been withdrawn.

5. A new sheath should be used every time lovemaking takes place.

The Rhythm Method

Uses

Limited effectiveness.

Information available from:
    Catholic Advisory Marriage Council,
    Clitherow House,
    15 Lansdowne Road,
    London W11 3AJ.

The Vaginal Diaphragm

Uses

Useful alternative for those who cannot or should not take the pill. Effective but onus is on the user to take correct action before coitus. Difficulties where there is prolapse or poor vaginal tone.

Types

Soft coil spring diaphragm in 5 mm graded sizes from 50–100 mm (most women 70–85 mm size).

Cervical cap.

Vault cap.

Fitting

A set of fitting rings should be obtained from the manufacturer, e.g. Ortho or London Rubber.

1. The diaphragm fits across the vault of the vagina from the posterior fornix to the retropubic space, thus covering the cervix.

2. The largest comfortable size should be fitted to help cope with changes in vaginal size and shape during coitus.

3. Can be inserted with the dome up or down (usually up) and the direction of the cervix is immaterial.

4. Correct size will fit comfortably without distending the vaginal walls and the anterior rim will not descend below the lower edge of the symphysis (even when the patient strains down).

5. Once correctly fitted the patient should be unaware of its presence.

6. At the first visit a practice diaphragm is fitted and after a 1–2 week trial the patient leaves it in place for a few hours before coming for a final fitting.

Advice to the patient

1. Always use a spermicidal cream with your diaphragm.

2. Put your diaphragm in at any convenient time before intercourse.

3. Check the diaphragm is covering the cervix.

4. If you have intercourse more than 3 hours after inserting the diaphragm then use more cream or a pessary (without removing the diaphragm).

5. Do not remove the diaphragm for at least 6 hours after intercourse. Do not leave it in for more than 24 hours.

6. After use, clean the diaphragm gently in soap and water. Rinse and dry thoroughly.

7. Mention – if weight gain or loss of more than 7 lb then come for check.

Follow-up

Attend with diaphragm in position.

If fitted in puerperium, after a vaginal operation or before regular coitus then see in 6 weeks to 3 months, otherwise yearly check for fitting and possible replacement.

The IUCD or Coil

Uses   Alternative to the pill for parous women.

Eliminates risks in poorly motivated couples.

Types   Larger plastic devices (Lippes, Saf T, etc.)
O greater side effects

O do not need to be changed.

Smaller copper devices.

O fewer side effects

O need to be changed every 2–5 years.

Contraindications   Menorrhagia, abnormal uterine bleeding, history of severe anaemia.

Recent acute pelvic inflammation or acute cervicitis.

Past history of ectopic pregnancy.

Congenital or acquired abnormalities affecting the size or shape of the uterus.

Nulliparity (unless will accept no other method and understands the risk of pelvic inflammation leading to possible infertility).

Insertion   Skill in insertion techniques should be gained at courses run by the Joint Committee on Contraception.

Advice to patient

1. The coil is effective from the moment it has been fitted.
2. Mild cramping pains may occur after fitting and perhaps with the next few periods.
3. Your next few periods may well be heavier with some intermenstrual bleeding. Do not worry about this.
4. Some coils may be expelled and it is worth checking yourself for the threads after your first three periods.
5. Mention – pregnancy risk (2–3%).
   – possible side effects.

Follow-up   See at 6/52 or 12/52, and then at 12/12 and 24/12 for check speculum/VE.

Possible side effects   Pregnancy with coil *in situ* (N.B. MAY BE ECTOPIC).

Pelvic infection.

Abdominal cramp and dysmenorrhoea.

Menorrhagia.

Perforation.

Notes

1. Remove by pulling threads, with sponge forceps, downwards in direction of long axis of the cervix. Unless pregnancy is desired, remove during the menstrual period.

2. If thread is lost — ultrasound or X-ray pelvis to check position; refer.

3. If pregnant — consider removal of IUCD as soon as possible. If will not come out or threads cannot be found, refer immediately to a gynaecologist.

4. An IUCD can be fitted up to 5 days after the predicted date of ovulation to provide a very effective means of postcoital contraception.

5. At the menopause the IUCD should be removed 12 months after the last period.

Sterilization

○ In either partner is likely to be safer and more effective than using any reversible method for the same number of years.

○ Must be emphasized to the couple that for all practical purposes the procedures are irreversible.

○ Must be a full measure of counselling about medical and social factors and their implication for the future.

○ If all else is equal, vasectomy is preferable to female sterilization as it is easier to perform and safer.

Termination of Pregnancy

Though not strictly a method of contraception, termination is a necessary back-up facility while other methods have a greater or lesser risk of failure attached to their use. The role of the GP is to act as counsellor and then to make a referral to an NHS hospital or private clinic if termination is indicated.

The Abortion Act (1968)

Two medical practitioners must certify (on form HSA1) that a termination is necessary for one of the following reasons:

1. That continuing the pregnancy involves risk to the mother's life or of physical or mental injury greater than if the pregnancy were terminated.

2. That continuing the pregnancy involves a risk of mental or physical injury to existing children greater than if the pregnancy were terminated.

3. That there is a substantial risk that the child may be born with a serious mental or physical handicap.

Note

○ If a GP has a conscientious objection to termination it is reasonable to offer the patient the opportunity to consult another doctor.

○ In some areas terminations are difficult to obtain under the NHS. The private sector's response and medical standards are more predictable.

○ The earlier the termination is performed the lower the likelihood of complications. Carried out before 12 weeks the operation is generally a minor and very safe procedure.

A2 Antenatal Care

More than 98% of deliveries now occur in hospital. General practitioners provide total care for less than 20% of all pregnancies but shared care in most of the others.

Aims

1. To provide the mother with a healthy, full term baby and rapid recovery after a normal delivery.

2. To facilitate the live birth of a normal baby, free of congenital or developmental damage.

3. To help both mother and father to achieve the knowledge and capacity to provide for the physical, emotional and social needs of the baby.

Preconception care

Healthy women normally have healthy babies. Preconceptional care tries to ensure:

○ Any existing medical condition is under the best possible control, e.g. heart disease, haemoglobinopathies, diabetes, hypertension. Referral to a physician with a special interest may be necessary.

○ Any previous obstetric problems are carefully assessed, e.g. perinatal death, congenital abnormality, previous low birth weight, late pregnancy complications. Referral to a geneticist or obstetrician may be helpful.

○ Any hereditary disease risks are carefully assessed, e.g. conditions like haemophilia and muscular dystrophy when tests on the mother may identify her as a carrier. Refer to geneticist before conception if at all possible.

○ The woman is as fit as possible before conceiving
  - immune to rubella
  - free from sexually transmitted diseases
  - not smoking (partner also)
  - drinking as little alcohol as possible
  - taking regular physical exercise
  - as (unnecessarily) unstressed as possible
  - not losing weight (or too overweight) and eating three balanced meals a day.

Consultation plan

Initial booking – as early as possible	8–12 weeks
4 weekly until	28 weeks
2 weekly from 28 weeks to	36 weeks
Weekly thereafter to	Term
6 weeks after delivery	Postnatal

Shared care may alternate with hospital visits or hospital may see at two or three set times with GP doing the bulk of the antenatal care.

The Team

Antenatal clinics in general practice provide opportunity for productive co-operation between health visitor, midwife and GP.

The **health visitor** should be involved from early in pregnancy both to develop her own patient contacts and to carry out her vital role in health education.

The **midwife** should also be involved with any patients booked for GP maternity unit or home delivery.

Prescribing in pregnancy

○ Drugs can produce adverse effects on the fetus throughout the whole of pregnancy.
○ All drugs are capable of producing toxic effects to some degree so caution is required when prescribing to any woman of childbearing potential.
○ Drugs account for only 1–5% of severe congenital malformations but there are no reliable methods for predicting teratogenicity in man.
○ If the mother's health demands that drug treatment should be given then it should not be withheld merely because of pregnancy. The effects of the illness may be more detrimental to the fetus than the effects of the drug, e.g. poorly controlled epilepsy.
○ If drugs are required during pregnancy then those which have been extensively used and shown to be normally safe are to be preferred to new drugs.
○ Low risk drugs include
  – penicillins, erythromycin stearate, cephalosporins, nalidixic acid
  – vaginal antifungal medications
  – antacids
  – iron
  – paracetamol
  – drugs for asthma
  – methyldopa, clonidine
  – metoclopramide
  – insulin
  – heparin
  – tricyclic antidepressants

Suspected rubella contact in early pregnancy

1. Make sure patient is pregnant and less than 16 weeks.

2. How strong is the history of contact? Has the patient clinical evidence of rubella (rash, cervical glands, joint pains)?

3. Has the patient previously had rubella?

4. Do rubella antibody titres
   - ○ if immune then no further action
   - ○ if non-immune
     - ○ repeat antibody titres in 1–2 weeks
     - ○ if rising titres or definite clinical rubella
     - ○ discuss risks of fetal abnormality and termination of pregnancy.

There is no clear evidence that human immunoglobulin given to women, who are suspected contacts or who actually contract rubella in early pregnancy, will protect the fetus.

The earlier in pregnancy the worse the damage and if rubella develops in the first 11 weeks then all infants will be affected; if at 11–16 weeks 50% will have defects.

Preconditions for home confinement

With so little opportunity for GPs and midwives to gain experience of home confinement, this option will remain available to only a very carefully selected group of women.

Preconditions include:

1. Careful selection of low risk patients.

2. Patient and partner both wish home confinement and are both aware of the possible increased risks (about 25% of patients booked for home delivery will be transferred to hospital care either before or during labour).

3. Willing, competent GP with adequate training and confidence in home delivery techniques.

4. Willing, competent district midwife with adequate training and confidence in home delivery techniques.

5. An effective obstetric flying squad.

6. GP present at delivery to resuscitate baby, if necessary.

NB. If a woman insists on a home confinement (and she has the right to), the midwife is bound to attend her. The GP can refuse to accept her for obstetric care but if then called in an emergency, is obliged to attend. If contact has been lost with the patient and she has had no antenatal care then this may be worse than if the GP had gone along with her, however reluctantly, in the first place.

Indications for hospital delivery by specialist (rather than in GP unit)

1. Bad social history.
2. Primiparae.
3. Fourth or subsequent delivery.
4. Age alone regardless of parity, i.e. over 35 years.
5. Previous third stage abnormality.
6. All major medical disorders.
7. Multiple pregnancy.
8. All malpresentations.
9. Bad obstetric history.
10. Disproportion – actual or suspect.
11. Previous Caesarean Section, myomectomy or hysterotomy.
12. All hypertensive states.
13. Prematurity and history of premature labour.
14. Rh negative women with antibodies.
15. Gynaecological abnormality.
16. History of infertility.
17. Gross obesity.

Indications for prompt hospital referral during antenatal care

Early in pregnancy

1. History of CNS abnormality: discuss and refer for alphafetoprotein and amniocentesis.
2. Mother over the age of 40 discuss and then refer for test of fetal chromosomal pattern to exclude mongolism.
3. Clinical rubella or rising rubella antibody titre.
4. IUCD *in utero* (may be ectopic pregnancy).
5. Hyperemesis gravidarum.
6. Medical disorders, e.g. anaemia, diabetes, renal or heart disease.
7. Hypertension.
8. History of recurrent abortion.
9. Large for dates.

Later in pregnancy

1. Antepartum haemorrhage (bleeding after 28 weeks).
2. Malpresentations after 32 weeks, e.g. breech for external cephalic version.
3. Small for dates.
4. Large for dates.
5. Pre-eclampsia.
6. Suspected intrauterine death.
7. Development of diabetes or jaundice.

Specialist investigations

Ultrasound scanning

Most units now have real-time ultrasound B scan machines and either scan all women routinely or have a 'low threshold' for ordering scans. The Royal College of Obstetricians and Gynaecologists believes scanning is without adverse effect on mother and fetus.

○ Before 12 weeks can diagnose missed abortion, multiple pregnancy, occasional fetal abnormalities.
○ Can measure gestational age (crown–rump length) with an accuracy of + or − 5 days. Serial scans are more accurate and reliable than a single scan.
○ At about 18 weeks a normal scan can reassure the mother in cases of high alphafetoprotein and can reduce the number of amniocentesis procedures that need to be performed.
○ Third trimester scans can measure growth; locate the placenta; and diagnose fetal abnormalities such as polycystic kidney, hydrocephalus, duodenal atresia.

Alphafetoprotein screening

○ Blood is best taken at 16–18 weeks (not before 16).
○ Picks up 80–90% of fetuses with open spina bifida and anencephalus.
○ Couples must understand that a normal result does not guarantee a normal fetus.
○ Really only worthwhile doing in patients who would consider termination should the result prove to be positive.

Amniocentesis

○ Should be offered to all pregnant women over the age of 36.
○ Can pick up chromosomal abnormalities, e.g. Down's syndrome, open neural tube defects (fluid alphafetoprotein levels measured) and male fetuses at risk of a sex-linked disorder, i.e. if risk of haemophilia would show if fetus was male but not whether that male would actually get haemophilia.
○ Risk of spontaneous abortion in 1% of cases.
○ Does not guarantee a normal fetus.
○ Should not be carried out unless termination would be considered should an abnormality be discovered.

Initial examination (8–12 weeks pregnant)

Practice staff

Fill in form FP24   FP24/A.

Fill in personal details on co-operation card.

Weight.

Urinalysis for albumin and glucose.

BP.

Fill in forms for antenatal (tests may be carried out at hospital)
- ○ Hb
- ○ AB0 and Rhesus
- ○ Rubella antibodies
- ○ V.D.R.L.

Electrophoresis for abnormal haemoglobins in women of African or Indian extraction and Mediterranean stock.

MSU.

Doctor

Full medical history.

Menstrual history.

Calculate EDD.

Past gynaecological history.

Past obstetric history.

Physical examination including breasts and ? vaginal examination.

Anti-smoking propaganda if appropriate.

Pro-breast feeding propaganda.

Decide form and place of antenatal care and delivery.

Problem check list (see page 31).

All details filled in on co-operation card.

From 12–28 weeks

Practice staff

Weight.

BP.

Urinalysis for albumin and glucose.

Doctor

Fundus.

Check EDD.

Problem check list (see page 31).

Is alphafetoprotein screening to be arranged?

Is amniocentesis indicated?

Are iron or vitamin supplements required?

N.B. In pregnancy the Hb level cannot be taken as an absolute index of iron status because of the rate at which haemodilution occurs. Levels of 10.0 g/dl or less should raise suspicions of iron deficiency though mean cell volume (MCV) and mean cell Hb (MCH) levels should also be taken into account.

MCH (pg)	MCV (fl)	Interpretation
⩾26	80–105	Physiological
⩽25	60–78	Iron deficiency
21	65	? Thalassaemia trait
⩾28	⩾100	Folate deficiency

From 30 weeks onwards

Practice staff

Weight.

BP.

Urinalysis for albumin and glucose.

Encourage care of breasts.

Check iron, folic acid administration.

Arrange for parentcraft, relaxation classes, etc.

Doctor

Fundus.

Confirm fetal position.

Fetal heart if indicated.

Check EDD.

Problem check list (see page 31).

Is there any evidence of pre-eclampsia, intrauterine growth retardation or any other abnormality?

Are the booking arrangements still appropriate?

Also at 30 weeks	Check Hb, Rh antibodies if appropriate.
at 36 weeks	Check Hb, Rh antibodies if appropriate. Engagement of the head in primips.

Postnatal examination (6 weeks after delivery)

Practice staff

Weight.

BP.

Urinalysis for albumin and glucose.

Send off completed form FP24   FP24/A.

Doctor

Examine pelvis.

Examine breasts, if indicated.

Cervical smear, if indicated.

Contraception.

Problem check list (see below).

? follow-up, e.g. bacteriuria and investigate further.

Complete form FP24   FP24/A.

Complete form FP1001, 1002 or 1003 if appropriate.

Enquire about baby's progress and arrange to see at children's clinic.

Problem check list   Enquire about Work

Diet

Sex

Management of other children in family

Anxieties   ○ having a baby
○ hospital delivery
○ caring for baby
○ possible malformation of baby

Depression

Genetic counselling

A3 Child Care

Women in the reproductive age group and children below the age of 5 consult their GPs on average about five times per year. Many consultations are for preventive procedures and are an extension of antenatal care.

Aims

1. To establish **immunity** against specified infectious diseases.

2. To **detect and prevent** certain other diseases and problems before irreparable damage occurs.

3. To facilitate **growth and development** to the infant's optimal potential.

4. To provide a basis for **lifelong emotional stability;** especially through a loving relationship within the family.

Immunization

Vital to get full uptake from preventive viewpoint and also to maximize practice income. Special weekly clinic run by practice nurse or health visitor is best, but remember doctor is responsible for ensuring his staff are fully competent.

Age/sex register is valuable in ensuring no one is forgotten.

Developmental assessment

Intensive developmental screening is still of unproven value and the subject of much argument. However there can be no argument about the presumption that every GP should take every opportunity of appreciating the capabilities of normal infants and children. Thus, at any consultation, he can look for and recognize defects outside the range of normal.

There is little doubt some potentially remediable disorders of childhood can be picked up simply by non-invasive examination, e.g. congenital dislocation of the hip, maldescent of the testes, deafness, squint, decreased visual acuity.

The Handbook of Preventative Care for Pre-school Children

(GMSC/RCGP; October 1984) and child health record cards may be obtained from either

The Secretary,
General Medical Services
  Committee
BMA House,
Tavistock Square,
London WC1H 9JP.

or

Head of Information Services,
Royal College of General
  Practitioners,
14 Princes Gate,
Hyde Park,
London SW7 1PU.

Routine Preventive Care in the first 14 years of Life

Consultation plan

Age	Doctor	HV or Practice staff	Present DHSS immunization schedule
Birth	Hospital		
2–3 weeks		X	
6 weeks	At postnatal		
3 months		X	1st Triple* plus polio
$4\frac{1}{2}$ months		X	2nd Triple* plus polio
7 months	X		
$8\frac{1}{2}$–11 months		X	3rd Triple* plus polio
15 months		X	Measles
18 months		X	
2–$2\frac{1}{2}$ years	X		
$4\frac{1}{2}$ years	X	X	Diphtheria, tetanus plus polio
11–13 years		X	BCG for tuberculin negatives
10–13 years		X	Rubella (girls only)
15–19 years		X	Tetanus toxoid plus polio

* [1] If pertussis is not wanted or contraindicated then give diphtheria and tetanus.

[2] In event of whooping cough outbreak can give 'crash' regime of 3 doses of triple at monthly intervals from age 3 months.
A diphtheria/tetanus booster then has to be given at 12–18 months.

[3] Infants whose basic course of triple or polio vaccine has been interrupted should be given a single additional dose later in infancy (or two doses where only the first dose of the basic course has been given) regardless of the time elapsing between the initial and subsequent doses.

[4] Current practice for institution of immunization of prematurely born infants is to ignore gestational age and give immunizations at the usual chronological age, i.e. start triple and polio at 3 months of age.

Available vaccines

TABLE 1		
Live attenuated	**Inactivated/killed**	**Toxoid**
Polio (oral)	Pertussis	Tetanus
Measles	Typhoid	Diphtheria
Rubella	Cholera	
BCG	Influenza	
Mumps	Polio	
Yellow fever	Hepatitis B	
Chickenpox	Rabies	
	Anthrax	

Contraindications

TABLE 2a	Contraindications to inactivated/killed vaccines and toxoids
Vaccine/toxoid	**Contraindications**
Diphtheria	Persons over 10 unless Schick-positive
Tetanus	Booster dose within the past year
Pertussis	
Absolute	Acute febrile illness (postpone until recovered) History of any severe local or general reaction to a preceding dose History of cerebral irritation or damage in the neonatal period Infant suffered from fits or convulsions
Relative*	Parents or siblings with history of idiopathic epilepsy Children with developmental delay thought to be due to neurological defect Children with neurological disease
Influenza	Egg allergy Children below the age of 9
Typhoid, cholera rabies, anthrax	None

* For these groups of children the risks of vaccination may be higher than normal but the effects of whooping cough may also be more severe. The balance of risk and benefit should be assessed in each case

Contraindications
continued

TABLE 2b	Contraindications to **live vaccines**

GENERAL

A. Within 3 weeks of another live vaccine.

B. Pregnancy (unless risk of contracting the disease outweighs risk of fetal damage).

C. Acute febrile illness (postpone until recovered).

D. Immunological dysfunction, e.g. hypogammaglobulinaemia.

E. Malignant disease, e.g. leukaemia, Hodgkin's disease.

F. Steroid therapy.

G. Immunosuppressant therapy.

H. Radiotherapy.

SPECIFIC

Vaccine	Contraindications
Poliomyelitis	Diarrhoea and vomiting. PH serious adverse reaction to penicillin, neomycin, streptomycin or polymyxin.
Measles*	Active TB Allergy to polymyxin or neomycin History of anaphylactoid reaction to egg ingestion
BCG	Local septic conditions Chronic skin disease, e.g. eczema Heaf positive reactions (except Grade 1)
Rubella	Pregnancy and any possibility of pregnancy within 3 months following vaccination Allergy to neomycin and polymyxin Thrombocytopenia Rheumatoid arthritis
Influenza (live)	Below age of 9 years Allergy to egg protein

* Children with a personal history of convulsions, or a family history of idiopathic epilepsy in parents or siblings, should be given measles vaccine but only with simultaneous administration of specially diluted human normal immunoglobulin. This can be obtained from hospital pharmacies or The Blood Product Laboratory, Elstree (01-9536191)

Administration

TABLE 3				
Vaccine	Dose	Route	Adverse effects	Special Notes
Triple (Diph/Tet/Pert)	0.5 ml x 3	i.m. or deep s.c.	Transient local erythema and tenderness. Restlessness and irritability in 24 hours post vaccination. Occasional screaming fits. Rarely encephalopathy.	Joint Committee estimates 1 case of permanent brain damage per 100 000 children fully immunized. 75% of these cases have symptoms within 24 hours. Do not give to children over the age of 6 years.
Poliomyelitis Sabin	3 drops x 3	oral	Rarely vaccine related paralysis in recipients or contacts.	Joint Committee recommends that unvaccinated parents of a child being immunized are also offered immunization.
Measles	0.5 ml	i.m. or s.c.	Usually about 8th day with mild cough, cold, rash, pyrexia. Rarely high pyrexia and febrile convulsions. Encephalitis in 1 in 10^6.	Vaccine is quickly killed by either, alcohol or detergents. In child with chronic heart or lung disease or history of fits reactions can be reduced by concomitant injection of gammaglobulin into the muscle of the opposite limb.
BCG	0.1 ml	i.d.	Discharging ulcer. Rare severe local reaction with abcess.	Injection site best left uncovered to facilitate healing. May be given at same time as polio but 3 week rule applies to all other live vaccines.
Rubella	0.5 ml	s.c.	Mild symptoms of natural infection may occur on 9th day.	Only acetone, alcohol or ether should be used to swab the skin which must be allowed to dry before injection given.
Tetanus (booster)	0.5 ml	i.m. or deep s.c.	Transient local pain, tenderness and swelling especially in those who have previously been immunized against tetanus.	Give at 10–15 year intervals after primary course and pre-school booster.
Influenza (live)	0.5 ml	i.m. or deep s.c.	Mild URTI symptoms.	Must not come into contact with spirit.

KEEP VACCINES IN REFRIGERATOR BUT NOT FROZEN.

Special groups

TABLE 4

Anthrax	Workers at risk from animal products.
Influenza	Patients with chronic heart, respiratory or renal disease. Diabetes or other endocrine disorders. Patients in institutions, especially the young and old. Some nursing and medical personnel. High value business personnel (mass vaccination of all workers has not proved to be worthwhile).
Measles	Any child up to age 15 without immunity, especially at school entry.
Polio	Everyone in the neighbourhood of a case of the disease, a single oral dose regardless of state of immunity.
Rabies	Persons bitten or licked. Workers in contact with quarantined animals.
Rubella	Female schoolteachers, nursery staff, doctors and nurses in obstetric units, antenatal clinic staff – but antibody status should be determined first and pregnancy avoided for 12 weeks. Seronegative patients post partum.
Tuberculosis	Tuberculin negative students. Relevant hospital staff. Tuberculin negative contacts of known cases, including children of immigrants from TB areas.

Developmental Surveillance

General notes

1. Growth implies increasing size. Development implies increasing complexity.

2. Assessment of an infant's mental maturity is made from a study of his behaviour and reactions to standard stimuli from one month onwards. Comparisons can be drawn and give Development Quotient (DQ).

3. Achievement of a new stage is dependent on the growing maturity of the nervous system so development CANNOT be accelerated by outside stimulus.
On the other hand environmental factors and illness can retard it.

4. Development is made up of many fields and rate in each field can be very different.

5. Uniform retardation implies mental retardation or severe emotional deprivation, but retardation in a single field does not suggest mental retardation. It may be pattern for that child or due to lack of stimulation in that field, or due to organic disease, e.g. speech retardation from deafness.

6. Development rate is not constant. Learning is slow for the first 9 months then very fast.

Basic data

Place of birth
Date of birth
Complications
Birth rank (previous miscarriages/stillbirths)
Mother's age
Father's age
Significant family history

At Birth

At birth (by doctor/midwife conducting delivery, or paediatrician)

Check for:

Normal appearance with normal motor tone
Cataracts – red rash
Any deformity neck, arms and legs
Fontanelles
Down's syndrome
Micro-ophthalmia
Cleft palate/hare lip
Cardiac abnormality
Single umbilical artery
Abdominal mass (including renal)
Pilonidal sinus
Spina bifida
Hypospadias
Imperforate anus
Testes
Congenital dislocation of hips
Talipes
Femoral pulses

Hospital tests:

Guthrie Test and test for hypothyroidism

Record:

Familial history
Antenatal history
Apgar rating
Birth weight
Length $\big\}$ Record in percentiles
Head circumference

Discuss with paediatrician:

1. All babies who become clinically jaundiced in the first 24 hours.

2. Premature infants whose bilirubin has reached a level of 170 μmol/l.

3. Full term infants whose bilirubin has reached a level of 205 μmol/l.

4. Any jaundiced infant who has, in addition, lethargy, anorexia, vomiting or pale stools.

Apgar Scale: **Record score 60 seconds after delivery of baby**

The baby is rated 0, 1 or 2 for each of the five signs listed in the left-hand column. The overall score of 0 to 10 is the sum of the ratings of the five individual signs. Infants with a score of 4 or less need help with breathing.

Sign	0	1	2
Heart rate	Absent	Slow (below 100)	Over 100
Respiratory	Absent	Slow irregular	Good crying
Muscle tone	Flaccid	Some flexion of extremities	Active motion
Reflex irritability	No response	Grimace	Cry
Colour	Blue, pale	Body pink Extremities blue	Completely pink

The indications for active resuscitation are:

(a)   A baby severely depressed at birth (heart rate under 100, judged by auscultation, inspection or palpation for a few seconds only) or,

(b)   A baby not breathing properly 1 minute after delivery or later.

Motor Responses in the few weeks after birth

Ventral suspension:
1–3 weeks. Flexed elbow,
flexed knee, drooping of head.

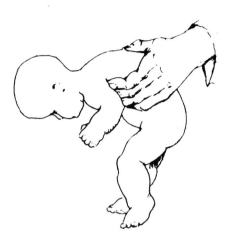

Sitting: First 4 weeks.
Completely rounded back.

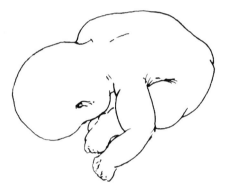

Supine position: First
4 weeks. Complete head
lag when pulled to
sitting position.

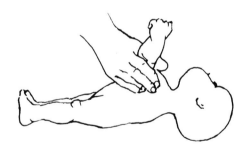

Prone position: 0–2 weeks.
Pelvis high, knees drawn
up under abdomen.

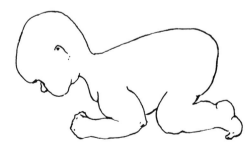

– After R. S. Illingworth

Motor Responses: 4–6 weeks after birth

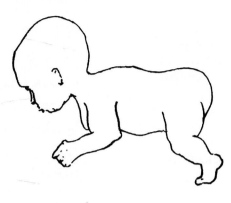

Prone position: 4–6 weeks. Pelvis still high. Intermittent extension of hips.

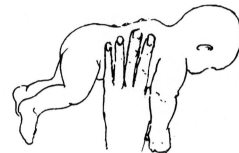

Ventral suspension: 6 weeks.

Sitting: 4–6 weeks. Rounded back. Head held up intermittently.

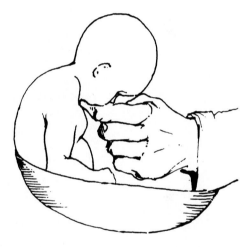

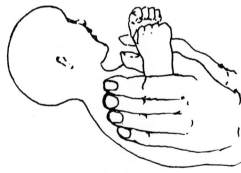

Supine position: 4 weeks.

Supine position: About 2 months. Considerable head lag when pulled to sitting but lag not complete.

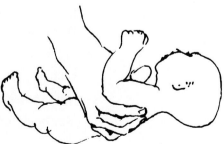

– After R. S. Illingworth

6 weeks

(preferably by GP and HV)

History
(unless
previously
recorded)

Antenatal
Natal
Postnatal

Present feeding (?breast; ?solids)

Mother's comments and queries

'Are you enjoying your baby?'

Examination

General appearance
Height/weight/skull (recorded on percentile charts)
Head shape
Ears
Eyes
Palate
Cardiovascular } cyanosis
heart sounds
femoral pulses

Chest
Abdomen
Hernial orifices } umbilical
inguinal

Genitalia
Hips (necessary to re-check)
Tone and reflexes
Arms and legs } missing or extra digits
talipes

Skin } naevi
seborrhoea/eczema
other skin blemishes

Discuss immunization and seek permission

Milestones

Check with mother or examine

Gross motor

Ventral suspension – head held up momentarily in same plane as rest of body.
Some extension of hips and flexion of knees. Flexion of elbows.

Prone – pelvis high, but knees no longer under abdomen.
Much intermittent extension of hips. Chin raised intermittently off couch. Head turned to one side.

Pull to sit – head lag considerable but not complete.

Held in sitting position – intermittently holds head up.

Held standing – no walking reflex. Head sags forward.

May hold head up momentarily.

Hands

Often open. Grasp reflex may be lost.

General understanding

Smiles at mother in response to overtures.

Vision

Eyes fixate on objects. They follow moving persons. In supine – looks at object held in midline, following it as it moves from the side to midline (90 degrees).

Hearing

Alert to sound.

Significant findings	Major anxiety in mother. Restricted abduction of the hip. Unusually large or small head. Excessive head lag and pulling to the sitting position. Asymmetry of tone. Delayed visual response.
Teaching topics	Management of minor illnesses. Safety in the home. 'Talk to your baby'.
Plans	Outline arrangements proposed for abnormalities found. Discuss immunization and seek permission. Appointment card for next check.

Motor Responses: 8–14 weeks

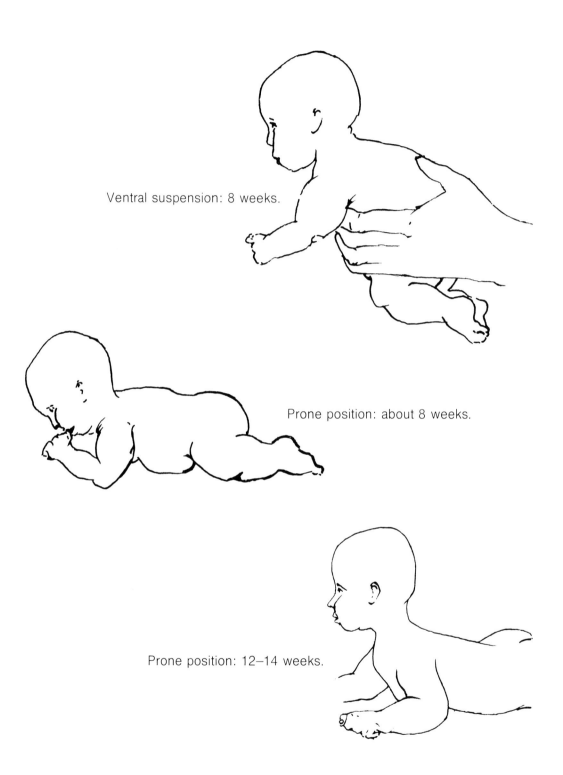

Ventral suspension: 8 weeks.

Prone position: about 8 weeks.

Prone position: 12–14 weeks.

– after R. S. Illingworth

7 months

7 months: (Examination by GP)

History

Mother's comments and queries
'Are you enjoying your baby?'
Any illnesses since last examination
Is baby happy?
Sleep pattern
Appetite
Feeding (breast to what age? solids started?)
Change in family circumstances
Does mother go out to work? Hours worked/week
Does baby go to nursery/child minder?
Check immunizations given and previous recommendations.

Examination

Length/weight/skull circumference (recorded on percentile charts).

Check
(a) Sit/stand/crawl – with/without support
(b) Grasp 1'' brick – what does he do with it?
(c) Hearing – (distraction test)
(d) Squint – refer now if in doubt
(e) Hips – refer now if in doubt
(f) How does child respond to examination?
(g) Heart sounds
(h) Femoral pulses
(i) Herniae – inguinal
              – umbilical
(j) Genitalia

Milestones

Check with mother or examine

Speech/hearing
Makes four different sounds.
Turns head to sound below level of ear.

General understanding
Looks for a fallen object.
Attracts attention by cough or other method.

Gross motor
Rolls from front to back.
Bounces if held standing.
Sits on floor for few seconds without support.

Hands
Feeds self with biscuit.
Drinks from cup.

Significant findings

Major anxiety in the mother.
Limited abduction of the hip.
Head circumference more than 2 standard deviations from the mean.
Abnormal posture.
Squint or nystagmus or failure to fixate.
Failed hearing test.
Delayed social/language development.

Teaching topics   Home safety.
Sleep independently.
Appointment card for next visit.

18 months

18 months: (examination by HV)

History

Mother's comments and queries
Any illnesses since last examination
Is baby happy?
Sleep pattern
Appetite?
Changes in family circumstances
Does mother go to work? (hours worked)
Does baby go to nursery/child minder?
Mother's opinion of speech development
Toilet training: clean by day/night
                 dry by day/night
Check immunization given and previous recommendations.

Examination

Height/weight/skull (recorded on percentile charts)

Review

Behaviour
Speech
Walking
Neuromuscular co-ordinafion (brick building, etc.)

Milestones

Check with mother or examine

Eyes
Check for strabismus, confrontation and light source.

Gross motor
Gets up and down stairs, holding rail, without help.
Walks up stairs, one hand held.
Walks, pulling toy or carrying doll.
Seats self on chair.
Beginning to jump (both feet).

Cubes
Tower of three or four.

Ball
Throws ball without fall.

Dressing
Takes off gloves, socks, unzips.

Feeding
Manages spoon well, without rotation.

Pencil
Spontaneous scribble. Makes stroke imitatively.

General understanding
'Domestic mimicry'. Copies mother in dusting, washing, cleaning.

Parts of body
Points to two or three (nose, eye, hair, etc.).

Picture card
Points to one ('Where is the . . . ?').

Book
Turns pages, two or three at a time.
Points to picture of car or dog.
Shows sustained interest.

Sphincter control
Dry by day, occasional accident.

Speech
Babble. Many intelligible words.

Simple formboard
Piles three blocks.

Significant findings

Major anxiety in the mother.
Not walking alone or walking with abnormal gait.
Squint.
Still mouthing.
Still casting objects.
Not vocalizing.

2–2½ years

2–2½ years: (examination by GP or HV)

History

Mother's comments and queries – her view of development
'Are you enjoying your child?'
Is baby happy?
Sleep pattern
Appetite?
Changes in family circumstances
Does mother go to work? (hours worked)
Does baby go to nursery/minder/play group?
Eating: knife–fork–spoon.
Toilet: clean by day/night
         dry by day/night
Can child dress itself?
Check immunizations given and previous recommendations.

Examination

Height/weight (recorded on percentile charts)
Dominant foot/hand/eye.

Review

Speech
Behaviour
Comprehension
Neuromuscular co-ordination.

Milestones

Check with mother or examine

Gross motor
Jumps off bottom step.
Goes up stairs, one foot per step, and down stairs, two feet per step.
Stands on one foot for seconds.
Rides tricycle.

Hands
Can help set table, not dropping china.

Cubes
Tower of nine.
Imitates building of bridge.

Dressing
Dresses and undresses fully if helped with buttons, and advised about correct shoe.
Unbuttons front and side buttons.

Pencils
Copies circle (from a card).
Imitates cross.
Draws a man on request.

General understanding
Knows some nursery rhymes.
Can name 8–12 subjects in a picture book.
Knows own first and last names.

Vision
1–8 rolling balls at 10.

Significant findings	Major anxiety in the mother.
	Failure to attain sphincter control.
	Abnormal gait.
	Squint.
	Failure to produce words and primitive sentences.
	Hyperactivity.
	Unusual bruising of the skin.
Teaching topics	Safety outside house.
	Sharing: discuss nursery/minder/play group.
	Appointment for next check.

$4\frac{1}{2}$ years

$4\frac{1}{2}$ years: pre-school (examination by GP)

History

Mother's comments and queries – her view of development
'Are you enjoying your child?'
Any illnesses since last examination?
Is child happy?
Sleep pattern
Appetite: Can he feed himself?
                   Use of knife–fork–spoon
                   Any fads?
Changes in family circumstances
Does mother go out to work?
Does child go to nursery/minder/play group/school?
Toilet: clean by day/night
              dry by day/night
Can child dress?
Check immunizations given and previous recommendations.

Examination

Height/weight (recorded·on percentile charts)
Dominant foot/hand/eye.
Vision: squint and acuity.
Hearing: Stycar sentences
                   audiogram if indicated.
Teeth

Review

Behaviour
Speech
Comprehension
Cardiovascular system
Limbs

Milestones

Check with mother or examine

Gross motor
Skips on both feet.
Heel/toe
Can walk on a straight line for at least four steps with gaps greater than 10 cm.

Vision
Stycar 9-letter test near and far vision.

Pencil
Copies triangle.

General understanding
Knows sex, age and address.
Distinguishes morning from afternoon
Compares two weights.

Colours
Names four.

Preposition (triple order)
'Put this on the chair, open the door, then give me that book'.

**Significant
findings**

Major anxiety in the mother.
Clumsiness.
Suspected defective vision.
Indistinct speech or stuttering.
Hyperactivity/behaviour problem.

Notes on the Use of Percentile Charts

Introduction

Body measurements for a given age vary from person to person. Reasons for variation include inherited constitution, dietary factors, emotional deprivation, and specific diseases.

Physical growth is one facet of total health, and must always be seen in this perspective. The correct goal is *optimal* growth within an optimal health situation. This will almost always mean less than *maximal* growth potential.

How to take measurements

Standing height (age 2 onwards).
Measurement without shoes, standing with heels, buttocks and shoulders in contact with an upright wall. Head looking straight forward with lower borders of eye sockets horizontal with ear openings. During measurement the child is told to stretch his neck to stand as tall as possible without the heels leaving the ground. The measurer applies gentle but firm traction upwards on the mastoid processes to assist this, and a right-angled block is slid down the wall to touch the child's head, a scale fixed to the wall being read to the nearest 0.1 cm.

Supine height (up to age 3).
Taken on flat surface with the child lying on back. One observer holds the child's head in contact with a board at the table top, whilst another straightens the legs, turns the feet at right angles, and slides a board in contact with the child's heels.

Weight
Take weight nude with empty bladder. If clothed subtract weight of clothes worn. Record to nearest 0.1 kg over the age of 6 months.

The use of percentiles

Distribution of measurements of children at each age is expressed in percentiles. A percentile refers to the position which a measurement would hold in any typical series of 100 children.

The 10th percentile is the value for the 10th in any 100 arranged in order, i.e. nine children of the same sex and age would be expected to be smaller than the measurement under consideration, while 90 would be larger. The 90th percentile similarly would show 89 children would be smaller and 10 would be larger. The 50th percentile marks the median position in the usual range. The 3rd and 97th percentiles mark the borderlines of the range of normal measurements. If a child falls below the 3rd or above the 97th percentile then in all probability he would be very much under or over weight or height respectively.

How to obtain a percentile position

Place a dot where the vertical age line intersects the horizontal line representing the reading taken.
Examples:
Boy age 10 years, weight 32 kg, percentile lies between 50th and 75th.
Boy age 10 years, height 134 cm, percentile lies between 24th and 50th.

Significance of percentiles

When periodic height–weight measurements are made, the percentile position can be compared with previous ones, and significant deviations recognized.

Under normal circumstances a child will maintain a similar position from age to age, that is on or near one percentile line or between the same two lines. When a sharp deviation or gradual shift from one percentile to another occurs, further investigation should be performed. An exception to this is in the pubertal years, when a child may drop to a lower percentile until he starts his growth spurt, rising rapidly whilst growing rapidly, and then dropping back to finish near the pre-pubertal percentile. Charts included in this book represent only average growth at given age, and take no account of intense pubertal growth.

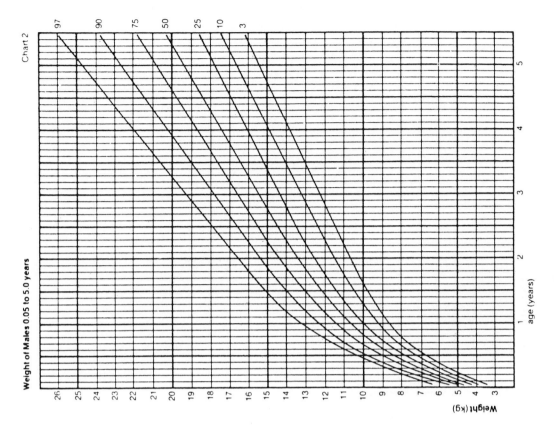

Weight of Males 0.05 to 5.0 years — Chart 2

Weight (kg): 3, 4, 5, 6, 7, 8, 9, 10, 11, 12, 13, 14, 15, 16, 17, 18, 19, 20, 21, 22, 23, 24, 25, 26

age (years): 1, 2, 3, 4, 5

Percentiles: 97, 90, 75, 50, 25, 10, 3

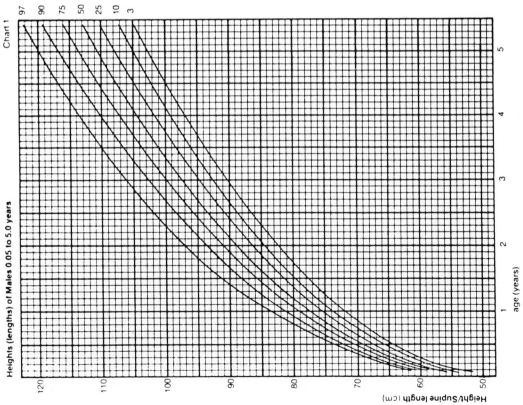

Heights (lengths) of Males 0.05 to 5.0 years — Chart 1

Height/Supine length (cm): 50, 60, 70, 80, 90, 100, 110, 120

age (years): 1, 2, 3, 4, 5

Percentiles: 97, 90, 75, 50, 25, 10, 3

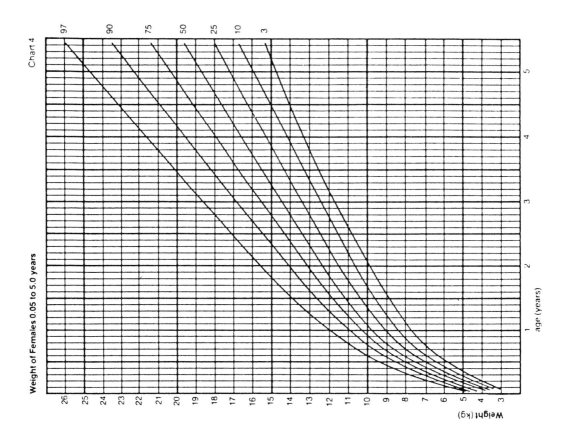

Weight of Females 0.05 to 5.0 years

Chart 4

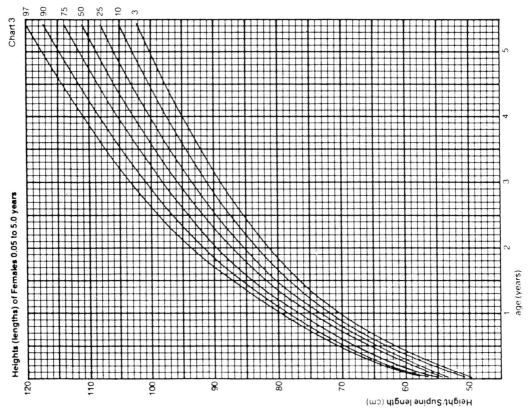

Heights (lengths) of Females 0.05 to 5.0 years

Chart 3

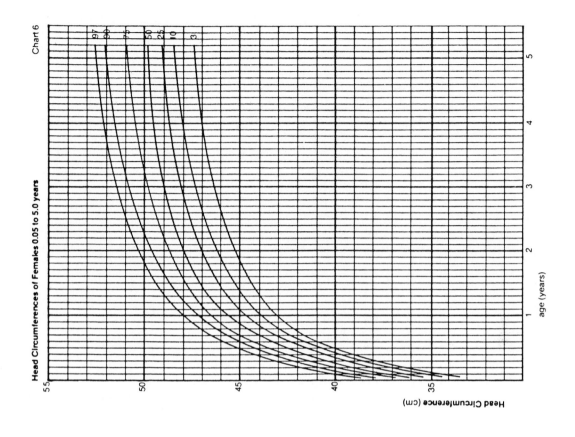

Chart 6

Head Circumferences of Females 0.05 to 5.0 years

Head Circumference (cm)

age (years)

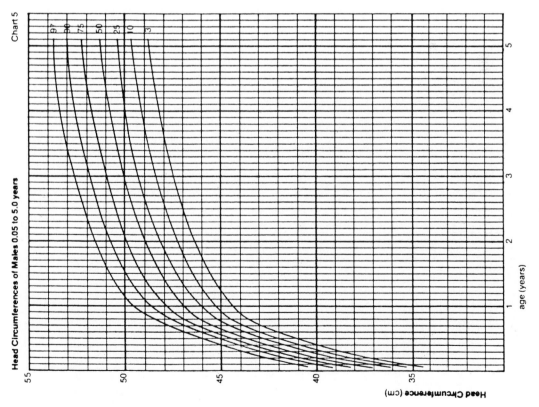

Chart 5

Head Circumferences of Males 0.05 to 5.0 years

Head Circumference (cm)

age (years)

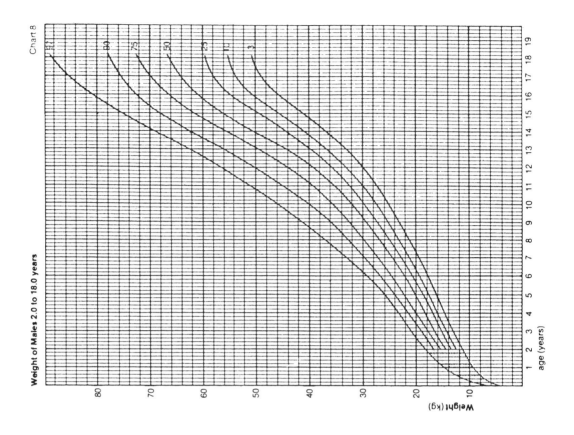

Heights (lengths) of Males 2.0 to 18.0 years

Chart 7

Height/Supine length (cm)

age (years)

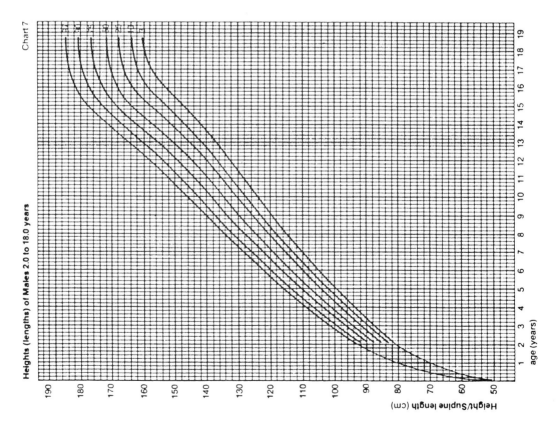

Weight of Males 2.0 to 18.0 years

Chart 8

Weight (kg)

age (years)

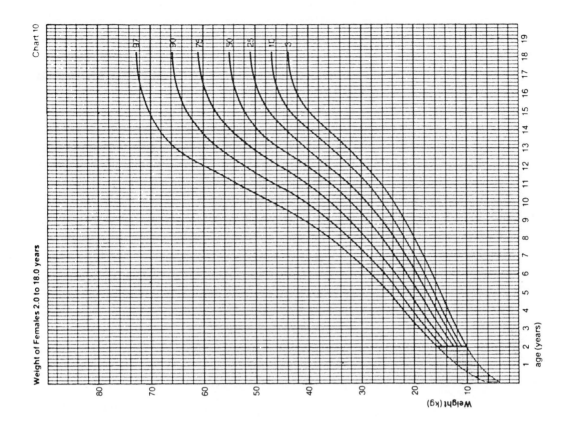

Chart 9

Heights (lengths) of Females 2.0 to 18.0 years

Height/Supine length (cm)

age (years)

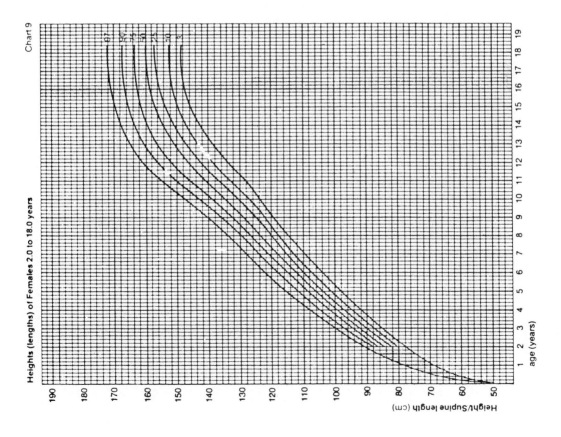

Chart 10

Weight of Females 2.0 to 18.0 years

Weight (kg)

age (years)

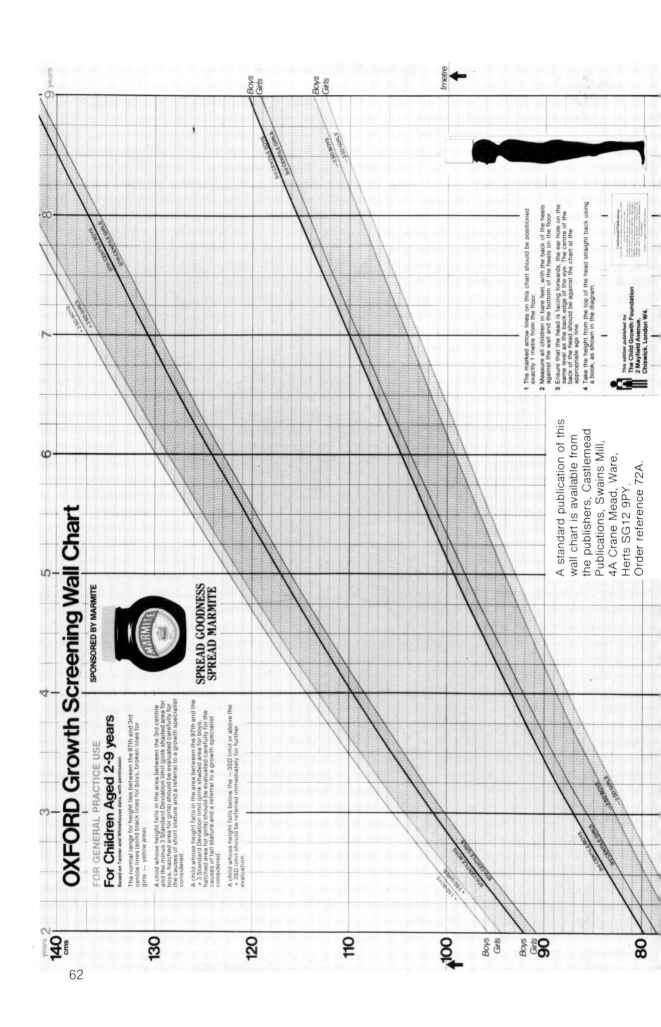

OXFORD Growth Screening Wall Chart

SPONSORED BY MARMITE

FOR GENERAL PRACTICE USE
For Children Aged 2-9 years

Based on Tanner and Whitehouse data, with permission.

The normal range for height lies between the 97th and 3rd centile lines (solid black lines for boys, broken lines for girls — yellow area).

A child whose height falls in the area between the 3rd centile and the minus 3 Standard Deviation limit (pink shaded area for boys, hatched area for girls) should be evaluated carefully for the causes of short stature and a referral to a growth specialist considered.

A child whose height falls in the area between the 97th and the + 3 Standard Deviation limit (pink shaded area for boys, hatched area for girls) should be evaluated carefully for the causes of tall stature and a referral to a growth specialist considered

A child whose height falls below the —3SD limit or above the + 3SD limit should be referred immediately for further evaluation.

SPREAD GOODNESS
SPREAD MARMITE

1 The marked arrow lines on this chart should be positioned exactly 1 metre from the floor.

2 Measure all children in bare feet, with the back of the heels against the wall and the bottom of the heels on the floor.

3 Ensure that the head is facing forwards, the ear hole on the same level as the back edge of the eye. The centre of the back of the head should be against the chart at the appropriate age line.

4 Take the height from the top of the head straight back using a book, as shown in the diagram.

This edition published for
The Child Growth Foundation
2 Mayfield Avenue,
Chiswick, London W4.

A standard publication of this wall chart is available from the publishers, Castlemead Publications, Swains Mill, 4A Crane Mead, Ware, Herts SG12 9PY. Order reference 72A.

A4   The Adolescent

Objectives

1. To advise and educate patient or relatives about normal development where this is in doubt.

2. To inform patient about possible hazards to health implicit in his lifestyle, and to encourage healthy modes of living while allowing for adequate and satisfying experimentation.

3. To encourage parents to accept the individual as he is at the time even if this is uncomfortable. Not to do so increases conflict and is likely to make problems worse.

3. To distinguish the rare cases of serious physical or psychiatric disease.

Problems

1. The most difficult may be to **establish an efficient and sensitive doctor–patient relationship.**

   The G.P. may be rejected as being identified too closely with parents, but adolescent may be unable or unwilling to change his doctor.
   'Will he laugh at me?'
   'Will he listen to me?'
   'Will he tell my parents?'

   There seems no reason to alter the ethical framework which governs every other consultation, i.e. what passes between adolescent and doctor is said **in confidence** and is respected by both as such.

   A major problem for adolescents is in gaining acceptance as individuals, whose attitudes and beliefs are as valid as those of anyone else. Much of what they stand for is dismissed or denigrated by parents and teachers and rebelliousness understandably follows. The doctor, whatever his own opinions, must not add to this problem. His aim should be to help the adolescent to build up his self-confidence and self-respect.

2. **Ignorance and rebelliousness may lead to poor use of services,** lack of self-care and subsequent problems, e.g.
   no contraception leads to unwanted pregnancy,
   excessive drinking or smoking leads to illness,
   unresolved emotional problems lead to parasuicide or breakdown.

3. **Poor education about illness and normality**
   may lead to frequent attendance for trivial complaints, and subsequent rejection by doctor
   or may lead to over-high expectations of what doctors can achieve and subsequent disappointment and rejection of doctor.

4. **The teenager experiences abrupt changes** in his life for which he has little preparation. There may be serious conflicts, e.g. between his parents' expectations and the lifestyle which he is experimenting with, alongside his peers. The adolescent's increasing need for privacy is very important and this applies particularly to sexuality and sexual experimentation. Even in the most well-adjusted, problem-free

families, it is unusual for a teenager to discuss his or her sexual activities with parents. It should not be expected. Sometimes teenagers will talk to doctors especially about contraception, but only if they feel they can be absolutely sure that confidentiality will be respected.

5. **The patient may be presented obliquely,** in his absence, by parents, with the request to "do something" about particular behaviour. Dealing with the guilt or anger of the referring person may be the only move possible. Parents should be encouraged to allow the youngster freedom to work out his own lifestyle even if this involves making mistakes. If the young person and the doctor think there is no medical problem, then the parents' pressure for referral, e.g. to a psychiatrist, must be resisted.

Normal abnormalities

○ Adolescent's anxieties must always be taken seriously and careful explanation given where appropriate. Never laugh them off.
○ Mastitis of puberty in boys is common and may be bilateral or unilateral. The boy must be specifically reassured that he is not changing sex.
○ Acne must be treated with enthusiasm and sympathy but beware of giving long term oxytetracycline with the contraceptive pill.
○ Striae are common and worrying to some.
○ Penile size may cause anxiety.

Smoking

○ Nearly all will try it, some will continue.
○ More likely to continue if parents smoke.
○ Difficult to persuade them not to, when so many adults do. Therefore probably better not to try and stick to straight information.
○ Smoking affects athletic performance – measure PFR and show how much it is reduced.
○ Smoking introduces risk to taking oral contraceptive.

Solvent abuse

○ Usual method is to put glue in a crisp bag and breathe the vapour (toluene). Sometimes aerosols are used and sprayed directly into the mouth. Practised mostly by males aged 12–15 years – rarely after 16 years. Causes intoxication similar to alcohol but shorter lasting.
○ Dangers from accidental anoxia from breathing from plastic bag, unconsciousness and inhalation of vomit; some toxic effects on brain and liver. Inhaling direct from aerosol much more dangerous than vapours from plastic bag.
○ Usually only a problem in children with social difficulties. The rest give it up quite soon without having taken any very serious risk.
○ May be safer than smoking or alcohol, if they must do something.
○ Important to reassure parents and try to make sure they do not overreact.
○ Examine social problems if indicated.

Drug addiction

○ Usually presented to doctor by parents after trouble with police or overdose incident.
○ GP's role usually confined to comforting and supporting family and being available as accepting friend for the addict, if he should ever seek one.
○ Medical treatment has no influence on outcome but factual information is useful – for instance how much more dangerous it is to inject heroin than to snort it and how much more dangerous it is to use barbiturates than anything, including heroin.
○ It is important not to prescribe especially barbiturates and Diconal but also tranquillizers, which are sometimes injected.

	○ Knowledge of local helping agencies should be available.
	○ Opiate addicts have 2½ times the risk of dying than others of their age, but 10 years later 50% are alive and well and off drugs with or without treatment.
Alcoholism	○ Heavy drinking now common in 16-plus age group.
	○ Useful to try to spot the potential alcoholic when young, as information given at this age may influence him to try to reduce drinking at a stage when it may not be too difficult.
	○ Once suspected, L.F.T.s including a γ-G.T. estimation may impress the youngster, if abnormal.
	○ Should be told that ability to think clearly, handle his job (or get one), drive a car, may all be damaged quite soon and that reaction times, physical strength, athletic and sexual prowess may be reduced.
	○ Information on helping organizations should be available.
	A heavy drinker is a man who drinks more than 50 units or a woman who drinks more than 25 units a week. A unit is ½ pint beer or 1 pub single spirits, or 1 pub measure sherry or 1 glass table wine.
Anorexia nervosa	○ Definition vague.
	○ Should be suspected in any girl who has marked loss of weight and **secondary** amenorrhoea.
	○ Mild cases are very common.
	○ The girl herself may present because of the amenorrhoea (never because of the weight loss), or parents or friends may come about her.
	○ Mild cases often respond to firm but friendly advice and frequent contact.
	○ Emphasis should be on: the fact that her periods have stopped shows that she is damaging her health by her dieting and must get her weight up enough to get the periods going again.
	○ It is pointless arguing about whether she is underweight.
	○ Some girls purge and some binge and vomit (bulimia). Exactly how the weight loss is achieved is really irrelevant.
	○ Treatment by psychiatrists is disappointing but severe cases have a high mortality and must be referred if possible to a specialist unit. If they can be kept alive they may make a spontaneous recovery.

Some statistics

Causes of death in the UK in 15–24 age group, per 100 000

All causes	52
Accidents	35
Neoplasms	7
Respiratory diseases	4
CVS	3
Other	3

Causes of morbidity: Annual consulting rates in 15–24 age group, per 1000

Respiratory infections	230
Mental illness	125
Skin disorders	120
Genito-urinary diseases	110
Accidents	95

Social morbidity

Up to 20% of youths under age of 20 are likely to appear in Court.
30 to 90% of youths interviewed admit breaches of the law.
(Moral – beware statistics!)

Methods of avoiding problems

Make confidentiality clear.
Treat adolescent as patient in own right, i.e. never accept consultation with relative present unless clinically indicated or patient wants it so.
Listen.
Educate.
Do not criticize or moralize.
Refer early if in doubt.

Important techniques/ knowledge

Legal responsibility and ages of consent.
Family planning: **all** methods.
Venereal disease: knowledge of presentation,
                             methods of diagnosis,
                             sources of help.
Antenatal care.
Counselling.
Services outside surgery for distressed teenagers, e.g.
     educational welfare
     counselling agencies
     employment advice
     social service agencies.

A5 Care of Adults

Scope and opportunities

Special features of general practice that should be utilized in planned care are:
- ○ frequent and regular contact between doctors and patients (average of 3–4 annual contacts).
- ○ long term care in a relatively small (2500 persons) and stable practice community.
- ○ scope for prevention, early diagnosis and long term care.

Objectives

To maintain lifetime records, to monitor health, and to make early diagnosis of disease from
- ○ regular recording of basic clinical data
- ○ information on personal habits and behaviour
- ○ information on the family.

Difficulties

No accepted programme of regular lifetime health maintenance in the NHS. Medical check-ups and screening exercises are complex, expensive and of uncertain value.

The standard NHS records are not designed for regular data recording.

Methods

Planned care for adults (and for other age groups) requires a programme that is meaningful and acceptable to the public and to doctors.

The **basic data** recorded must be simple, reliable and useful.

The **methods of recording** must be simple, cheap and easy to use and apply.

Records (based on current summary cards) must be simple to use and to analyse.

Record keeping

Good records are an essential aid to good practice. Achieving worthwhile records is a somewhat boring, repetitive and time-consuming activity and so it is often not accorded any real priority.

Good records are necessary
○ as an accurate *aide-mémoire* to remind the doctor about previous events and investigations,
○ to aid communication in group practices and within the practice team,
○ to help plan continuing care,
○ to allow the monitoring of long term illnesses and act as the basis for a recall system,
○ to permit the implementation of screening programmes,
○ as a useful teaching aid,
○ for medicolegal purposes,
○ to provide a data base for audit and research,
○ to help maximize practice income.

Minimum criteria

For adequate records the minimum criteria include

1. summary card with clinical, family, social data,

2. hospital letters and reports filed in chronological order (and, ideally, regularly pruned),

3. recording of long term medication independently of continuation notes.

Lloyd-George or A4

A4-sized records allow all hospital reports to be filed flat and provide more space for the writing of adequate notes. However conversion to them is costly in time and money and they also take up more storage space than conventional records.

The useful information that needs to be retained for any patient is small. The work involved (filleting, summarizing, using special cards etc) in selectively retaining and clearly presenting information to make the Lloyd-George system work well equally needs to be carried out to make A4 records work well.

Getting records into order

This is hard work. In most practices virtually every patient envelope will need remedial surgery to trim off surplus information and to organize the rest into an easily accessible and retrievable form.

Contents in date order

A mass of cards and letters that are in a hopeless jumble frustrates information access and is a barrier to good care. Putting paper into date order, trimming letters to size, removing obviously unnecessary paper (e.g. old blank cards, hospital letters saying 'patient did not attend'), renewing record envelopes, is not skilled work. Properly instructed ancillary staff can easily cope with the work involved as can students or other reasonably bright youngsters taken on specifically to help.

Pruning

Most pruning should take place as the summary card is compiled. Getting rid of unnecessary paper results in slimmer notes which
　are more useful medically,
　change the doctor's perception of the patient,
　are more easily handled by receptionists,
　save filing cabinet space.

Adequate records do not mean records retaining everything ever received about a patient no matter its importance or relevance. For medicolegal reasons one has to be reasonably selective about what is thrown away but there can be no excuse for keeping masses of follow-up letters or old investigation reports.

As a rule of thumb – most letters (some longer or more important ones can be retained or a note of the hospital and reference number kept on the summary card), nearly all investigation reports (a note can be made of results on the continuation card or summary card), and about 1 in 3 continuation cards (empty ones, ones with only 1–2 entries not worth recording elsewhere, totally illegible ones, records of totally trivial events of long ago), can be safely removed.

Remember, Family Practitioner Committees only keep records of dead patients for 2 years before completely destroying them.

Summarizing

Ideally every record should contain a clear summary of all important medical and social conditions on an easily identified summary card *(see illustration below)*.

To summarize a set of records, the GP should do the following.
○ Look through the continuation cards to note significant conditions like eczema, psoriasis, asthma, migraine, depression which are unlikely to be also recorded in the hospital letters. Also note trends of patient behaviour and significant social information.
○ Look through the hospital letters compiling a clear, precise summary and discarding letters and reports as their contents are noted. Insert significant practice diagnoses and social pathology into the appropriate chronological spot.

A thinnish envelope may take 2–3 minutes, a big fat one 20–30. Twenty-five records modernized a week would add up to 1000 or more a year.

Using records to improve patient care

Recording the consultation

For every consultation a brief record should be made covering

○ the problem presented

○ important positive and negative verbal and physical findings

○ description of condition or diagnosis

○ management plan

This should be legible, and important features such as the diagnosis or investigations may be highlighted in some way, e.g. by being written or ringed in red or green.

Monitoring repeat prescribing

An efficient repeat prescribing system can be used to monitor patients with chronic conditions and to ensure that those patients who have not been seen for a reasonable length of time can be asked to reattend. Essential elements include the following.

1. An up-to-date separate, easily identified repeat drug card in the record envelope.

2. A prominent space on the corresponding patient's repeat card showing when or after how many repeats the card is valid to *(see illustration, below).*

3. Careful scrutiny of the notes associated with invalid cards to see if the patient should be requested to attend for follow-up.

Using special cards

The use of special cards for long term problems can improve clinical care. Cards like the almost universally used antenatal co-operation card

1. collect relevant information together,

2. allow progress to be easily followed,

3. guide care along certain paths,

4. act as a reminder for certain regular, specified checks and investigations.

Other special cards can be used to help care for hypertensives *(see illustration below),* diabetics, epileptics, asthmatics, patients requiring family planning advice and so on.

Aiding prevention

Good records can act as a reminder for opportunistic screening. The front of the record envelope (and/or the summary card and the contraceptive record card) can be marked by colour-coded stickers which show, for example, when the last smear or BP was taken and when, by implication, the next one is due. The back of the record envelope can be reserved solely to record immunizations and so can be easily screened before any consultation to check if a jab is due.

This method of screening is cheap and is purely doctor-dependent with the flagged records acting as both the screening record and reminder. 90% or so of the practice population can be screened over a 5-year period and as easily rescreened over the next 5 years.

Summary of treatment card

MALE

SUMMARY OF TREATMENT CARD	
Surname	Ceeper
Forename(s)	Eileen
Address	71 Railway Approach
N.H.S. Number	Date of Birth 8/3/37

DATE	CLINICAL NOTES Para 2/1
1957	T + A
1961	Psychoneurosis → 1962 Thyrotoxicosis → Partial thyroidectomy
1965	Flare up thyrotoxicosis — carbimazole
1968	Radioiodine
1974	Smear — NAD + 81
1979	T₄ = 81 TSH = 8.2
1982	T₄ = 81 TSH = 7.5
1984	T₄ = 83 TSH = 13
1984	Divorced. Living with boyfriend
*	Now on thyroxine. Check thyroid function annually *

FP9A

Dd 8810139 2 675M 10/83 Ed (212290)

This record is the property of the Secretary of State for Social Services

DATE	CLINICAL NOTES

71

Repeat prescription card

<table>
<tr><td colspan="3">THIS CARD IS VALID UNTIL</td><td colspan="2">LAINDON HEALTH CENTRE
REPEAT PRESCRIPTION CARD</td></tr>
</table>

THIS CARD IS VALID UNTIL

Jan 83		
July 83		
Jan 84		
July 84		
Jan 85		

LAINDON HEALTH CENTRE
REPEAT PRESCRIPTION CARD

Surname   Forename(s)

Address _____

_____

Doctor _____

To get a repeat prescription you should put this card in the special box in the health centre

Prescriptions will usually be ready for collection 24 hours later.

Please DO NOT USE THE TELEPHONE unless there is an emergency.

A stamped addressed envelope should be supplied if you want the prescription posted to you.

This card is only valid until the date shown on the back.

AFTER THE LATEST DATE SHOWN ABOVE YOUR TREATMENT MUST BE REVIEWED BY THE DOCTOR
PLEASE REMEMBER TO ALLOW AT
LEAST 24 HOURS FOR US TO
PROCESS YOUR PRESCRIPTION
MONDAY TO FRIDAY OR
48 HOURS AT WEEKENDS   LHC 18

CURRENT TREATMENT

	DRUGS. STRENGTH. DOSE.	No:	DATE	DRUGS	DATE	DRUGS
1						
2						
3						
4						
5						
6						
7						
8						
9						
10						

DATE	BP	NOTES	?Fundi

NAME Frank Smith   **DOB** 18/6/40

Initial 1	180/110	2 175/105	3 175/105

BPS

Fam Hist Brothers ↑BP **RISK FACTORS**
Father + MI
Over wt X   Alcohol X   Personality   Likely to be
Smoking 10 a day   Exercise Regular   Type A Complier
                    Diabetes X   ↑Lipids X

ASSESSMENT

Wheezy? X   Chest pain? X   Cold extremities? X
Breathless? X   Gout? ✓

CVS EXAM:
FUNDI: Grade II   Femoral pulses X

INVESTIGATIONS

Urine Neg   ECG?   Lipids??
U/E NAD   LFT?   Glucose?
Uric acid NAD   IVP??

TRT AIM To get BP ≤ 140/90

ADVICE

Diet/Wt X   Alcohol X   Need for treatment X
Smoking Leaflet   Exercise ✓   LEAFLET given +
                                      benefit.

DATE	BP	NOTES	?Fundi
16/11/83	175/105	Atenolol 50 qs mane ㉘	See 2/52
30/11/83	155/95	No problems. Contd 50 qs mane ㉘	See 4/52
28/12/83	150/95	Atenolol 100 qs mane ㉘	See 1/2

73

Table of normal values

BIOCHEMISTRY
(serum or plasma)

Sodium	135–145 mmol/l	Total calcium	2.12–2.62 mmol/l
Potassium	3.5–5 mmol/l	Inorganic phosphate	0.8–1.4 mmol/l
Chloride	96–106 mmol/l	Total protein	60–80 g/l
Bicarbonate	23–29 mmol/l	Albumin	35–50 g/l
Urea	2.5–7 mmol/l	Globulin	20–40 g/l
Creatinine	60–130 μmol/l		
Urate	0.12–0.42 mmol/l		
Biliruben (total)	5–17 μmol/l	5–Nucleotidase	1–15 iu/l
Aspartate aminotransferase	5–40 iu/l	glutamyltransferase	0–60 iu/l ♂
Alkaline phosphatase	30–110 iu/l		0–40 iu/l ♀
Cholesterol	2.2–2.6 mmol/l	Triglyceride (fasting)	1.8 mmol/l
Glucose (fasting)	3.3–5.9 mmol/l	Glycosolated haemoglobin	5–9% of Hb
T4 (total)	55–144 nmol/l	TSH	1–5 miu/l
T4 (free)	10–30 pmol/l	T3	0.9–2.8 nmol/l
Acid phosphatase	0–13 iu/l	Amylase	70–300 iu/l

HAEMATOLOGY

Hb♂	15.5±2.5 g/dl	Hb♀	14±2.5 g/dl
RBC♂	5.5±1 × 10^{12}/l	RBC♀	4.8±1 × 10^{12}/l
PCV♂	0.47±0.07	PCV♀	0.42±0.05
MCV	85±8 fl	WBC	7.5±3.5 × 10^{9}/l
MCH	29.5±2.5 pg	Neutrophils	40–75%
MCHC	33±2g/dl	Lymphocytes	20–45%
Reticulocytes	0.2–2%	Monocytes	2–10%
Platelets	150–400 × 10^{9}/l	Eosinophils	1–6%
		Basophils	1%

Serum B_{12}	150–1000 ng/l	Serum iron	12–26 µg/l

Serum folate	2.5–12 µg/l	TIBC	45–70 µg/l
RBC folate	160–640 µg/l		

Bleeding time	1–7 min	Prothrombin time	10–14 seconds
Clotting time	10 min		

LUNG FUNCTION

FEV$_1$	♂3.5±1.5 l	♀2.5±1.0 l
FVC	♂4.5±1.5 l	♀3.5±1.0 l
PEFR	♂550±150 l/min	♀400±100 l/min

SEMINAL ANALYSIS

Normal range:
Volume	2.5–10 ml
No. of sperm	20 × 10^{6} per ml
Motility	70%
Morphology	60% normal forms

Overseas travel advice

Protective measures recommended depend on the countries to be visited, the length of stay and the conditions under which the traveller is expecting to live.

Condition	Notes
Pregnancy	After 35 weeks not allowed on long flights; after 36 weeks not allowed on short domestic flights.
Infectious diseases	During period of infectivity but does not include mild conditions like URTIs.
Respiratory disease	Pneumothorax (must have reabsorbed before flying); recent major chest surgery (within 3 weeks). **N.B.** Patients with chronic respiratory disease are at risk of hypoxia though they could be given O_2 for a short time on the plane.
Ear and sinus problems	Recent middle ear surgery; severe otitis media or sinusitis; and fixed wiring of the jaws. **N.B.** Special care is needed after stapedectomy.
Cardiovascular disease	Cardiac failure that is not in control; recent myocardial infarction (within 3–6 weeks); severe anaemia (below 7 g/dl); sickle cell disease (if homozygous mild hypoxia may cause sickling crisis).
Neurological disease	Recent stroke (within 3 weeks); recent air encephalopathy. **N.B.** Epileptics should increase their anticonvulsant therapy on the day of travel. Cerebral arteriosclerotics may become confused when hypoxic.
Psychiatric disorders	Can travel if well sedated and escorted.
Gastrointestinal disorders	Recent simple abdominal operation (within 10 days but longer if paralytic ileus had complicated recovery); recent peptic ulceration with haemorrhage (within 3 weeks). **N.B.** Ileostomists or colostomists should be advised to have extra bags and packing to hand and to take an antidiarrhoeal agent before flight.

For individual patients the medical department of the airline they are going to fly with is the best source of advice on fitness to travel and also about the facilities that are likely to be available for the disabled or ill traveller.

Sensible precautions

Condition	Advice on prevention
Water-borne infection	Always boil drinking water (chlorination with tablets is second-best), including that used for brushing teeth, and unpasteurized milk. Beware ice. Only drink well-known brands of bottled minerals (locally produced ones may not have been sterilized) and wipe the top well. The antibacterial low pH of carbonated drinks makes them a safer option. Never buy drinks, boiled tea or coffee possibly excepted, from local vendors.
Food-borne infection	Never eat food or ice-cream from street vendors. Eat fresh fruit and vegetables only if they can be peeled. Eat only food that has recently been cooked and is steaming hot. Meat especially should always be well done to avoid worm infestation. Avoid salads unless self-washed with sterilized water. Be very wary about shellfish and seafoods and avoid spicy foods.
Sunburn	Limit exposure to 15 minutes of hot summer sun initially (more if sunscreen lotions used) doubling time each day. Remember that one can still get sunburn while in water and through thin clothes. Sun-sensitive individuals should stay covered or in the shade as much as possible and use strong filtering lotions.
Prickly heat	Increase fluid intake; increase food salt. Wear light, loose cotton clothing; swim and shower frequently. Prevent copious sweating by reducing exertion.
Insect-borne infection	Keep well covered, long sleeved shirt and long trousers, after dark. If possible keep inside from dusk to dawn. Wire mesh over windows and mosquito netting may be necessary. Insect repellents can be applied to all exposed skin but must be regularly replaced. An insecticide aerosol spray should be kept handy. Avoid walking barefoot and check safety of all swimming areas before bathing.

Everyone should be encouraged to take out adequate medical insurance to cover both the cost of care abroad and the cost of travel home if still ill or injured.

Sexually transmitted disease	If in doubt, don't. If desperate, use sheath or diaphragm then wash or douche and micturate afterwards. **N.B.** Even after treatment abroad, anyone with symptoms or risk of VD should attend the special clinic.
Accidents	Treat alcohol with some respect. Do not pet stray animals. Pay due care and attention to local driving conditions. Treat cuts and abrasions very carefully. Maintain the highest standards of personal hygiene.

Immunization

To work out vaccine requirements for an individual traveller consider:

1. **Previous vaccination history** – so can decide whether needs boosters or primary courses (see table, below)

2. **Countries to be visited** – then look up recommended vaccinations needed (many medical journals have a chart containing the information).

3. **The time available to complete vaccine courses** – for those travellers who do not consult early enough to allow for optimal spacing of vaccines, a rapid scheme may be used though less effective immunity results, e.g.

   Day 1: Cholera, typhoid, oral polio, tetanus
   Day 5: Yellow fever (at special centre)
   Day 13: Cholera, oral polio
   Day 28: Typhoid, tetanus, oral polio

Vaccine programme information

Yellow fever	0.5 ml s.c. At special centre. One injection gives 10 years immunity. Not within 2 weeks of polio or gammaglobulin.
Typhoid	0.5 ml i.m. or deep s.c. then 0.1 ml i.d. after 4–6 weeks. 3-yearly boosters (0.1 ml i.d.) if still exposed to risk.
Cholera	0.5 ml i.m. then 0.2 ml i.d. after 1–4 weeks. 6-monthly booster (1 ml s.c.) if still exposed to risk.
Polio (live)	Three doses at 6 weeks then 6-month intervals. 5-yearly boosters. Not within 2 weeks of yellow fever or gammaglobulin.
Tetanus	0.5 ml deep s.c. or i.m. then at 4-week and 6-month intervals. 5–10-yearly boosters.
Gammaglobulin (HNIG)	5 ml deep i.m. protects against hepatitis A for up to 6 months. Give 4 days or so before travel.

Notes:

1. For all countries check if tetanus toxoid is needed.

2. Travellers to N. Europe, N. America, Japan, Australia and New Zealand require no particular immunization.

3. For overland travellers and those going to primitive regions use HNIG.

4. For travellers (not holidaymakers) to primitive regions give rabies vaccine.

5. Yellow fever vaccination is required for Central and S. America and Central, E. and W. Africa.

Malaria prophylaxis

Prophylactic drugs are needed even for a 1-day stay in a malarious area and should be started up to 1 week before travel and continued until at least 4 and up to 6 weeks after return to the UK. Tablets should not be given on NHS prescription but may be a private prescription or bought, without prescription, at the chemist (Fansidar, Maloprim have to be on prescription).

Changing patterns of resistance to antimalaria drugs mean that up-to-date information should be sought before advising patients. Journal travel guides are a good source but in cases of doubt specialist advice can be gained from:

DHSS, London: 01-407 5522 ext. 6711/6749
Ross Institute Tropical Hygiene: 01-636 8636

A6   Care of the Elderly

Objectives

1. To detect and distinguish disease from normal ageing, and where appropriate, treat.

2. To prevent avoidable misadventures (such as hypothermia, side effects of drug treatment).

3. To educate patients and relatives in the changing physiology and needs of the aged.

4. To preserve dignity and self-sufficiency for the patient within a framework of outside help which permits independence of mind if not of body.

5. To manage disease with knowledge of likely natural history and to appreciate that many problems of the elderly are non-curable. Nevertheless, that relief and comfort are always possible.

Problems

1. **Prevention.** Growing old is not preventable, but some medical problems of old age can be forestalled,
    e.g. painful feet ⟶ housebound lonely man ⟶ suicide or broken glasses ⟶ fall ⟶ fractured hip.

    The elderly are often reluctant to report disabilities as they want to see themselves as healthy and therefore independent. Often they leave problems, obvious to others, to deteriorate to a point where their health is permanently damaged, or where those surrounding them are angered or alienated by their apparent pig-headedness. This is worse in the poorer and less well-educated.

2. **Drugs and surgery** may need extra caution, if they are not to have unacceptably high physical, mental, social or ethical side effects. If things are going wrong, consider stopping a drug rather than starting another.

3. **Isolation** may be physical, social or emotional. Families may have moved away. Inflexible housing may create difficulties for the poorly mobile, and a need will not be detected until a crisis occurs.

4. **Bereavement** and grief are inevitable in married couples.

5. **Suicide,** rare, but more common in older men.

6. **Retirement** may be a crisis for a man or single woman. The abrupt transition may be like a minor death. 'I'm in the way', 'I'm on the scrap heap now'. The retired may have no activities, no role, no status, and worst of all no money. Many are fit to work still, and some find their way back to employment with satisfaction.

7. **Families** may need support to cope with a difficult relative.

8. **Resources** are limited and awareness and knowledge of what is available and useful makes for easier management.

9. **Multiple pathologies** are the rule. A choice has to be made on social and medical priorities.

Vital statistics	○ 15% of our present population are over 65 (i.e. 375 out of a practice of 2500). Of these, about 130 will be men and 245 women. Over 75, women outnumber men 3 to 1. Over 75, all problems of the elderly increase. ○ The elderly population will increase to a peak of nearly 20% at the end of the present century, when the number over 75 will almost equal those between 65 and 75. Consequently, the work load for general practitioners may double, as there is no evidence that there will be fewer health problems in the elderly. ○ Beyond 70 years old, many people cease to be able to lead an independent existence. Those unable to live at home without assistance increase from 12% in 65–69 age group to over 80% at the age of 85 years. ○ Morbidity and disability from chronic diseases in old age are higher in the lower social classes. ○ 94% of the country's pensioners live at home and are therefore cared for by general practitioners. 40% of consultations are with the elderly, who also have the highest consultation rates.
Organization	Combined care from practice team has to be backed up by hospital geriatric unit and social services.
Roles	**General Practice** **Doctor** supervises medical care and follow up, by routine method decided on as below, with preventive work based on knowledge of patients and relatives and backed up by age/sex register where applicable. **District Nurse** fully involved with continuing care of some patients, episodically with others. **Health Visitor** for preventive work and social visiting. **Receptionists** or other workers taking messages, encouraging, making arrangements for transport, etc and acting as the real first contacts with the practice. **District medical services** may provide screening clinics for the elderly, chiropody in the home or in clinics, audiology services, dentistry, occupational therapy or physiotherapy. **Geriatric unit** geriatrician for inpatient stay, clinics, domiciliary visits community geriatric nurse day unit **Psychiatrist** will advise and organize services on psychogeriatric problems. **Social services** Social worker Bathing attendant Meals on wheels Home help Occupational therapist Part III accommodation Day Centre for special needs **Terminal care** – (see subsection A7).

Follow-up

Regular follow-up by GP for selected patients. Check and visit (nurse or health visitor) non-attenders.

Visiting List
At Risk Register
List Patients Unable To Attend Surgery (PUTA)
Age/Sex Register
District Nurse/Health Visitor case load
Referrals from Social Services/District medical services

Possible regular follow-up methods include:

1. Monthly visits by district nurse with yearly full check-up by doctor

2. Car clinics – patients brought by practice transport or ambulance to the surgery.

3. Day unit attendance

4. Nurse questionnaire and check list.

5. Regular visits by doctor

6. Survey to discover needs which have not been met – can they feed, wash, dress, keep warm, move about in or outside, have they outside support or surveillance? Drugs, diet, dressings.

Check list

Possible problems

1. Can they get out?

    Heart failure?
    Incontinence?
    Fear of traffic or muggers?
    Housing – lifts or stairs?
    Cheap travel?
    Wheel chairs or walking aids?

2. Can they get around the house?

    Arthritis or bone pain?
    Immobility – day centre or physiotherapy for walking practice?
    Painful feet – chiropody?
    Occupation therapy – aids for daily living?

3. Can they wash and dress?

    Specific handicaps and specific aids?
    Bathing attendant?
    District nurse?
    Early morning anti-inflammatory for pain and stiffness?

4. Are they feeding adequately?

    Beware single and widowed, especially men
    Meals on wheels?
    Home helps for shopping?
    Dentures?

5. Are they warm?	Heating system and ability to pay bills? Prompt repair of vandalism? Prophylaxis of hypothermia, especially in Parkinsonism? Incontinence? Immobility?
6. Have they got enough money?	Social worker/health visitor? Attendance allowance? Rent and rate rebates? Holiday schemes with cheap travel? Death grant?
7. Can they keep clean?	Incontinence appliances and laundry service? Home help? Local authority disposal of large items
8. Are they safe?	Fire prevention – eliminate dangerous devices Lighting? Loose carpets?
9. Can they communicate?	Telephones? Whistle? Wax in ears? Hearing aids? Speech therapy after stroke? Dentures?
10. Are they happy?	Depression in old age? Loneliness: consider groups, pubs, neighbours Local schemes for visiting or day centres? Special aids – e.g. for blind? TV/radio? Holiday schemes? Neighbourhood schemes, or practice-based groups? Advice on incontinence and sexual matters?
11. Have they got the right medicines?	Clear labelling and instructions, written if possible. Access to GP services = flexible enough appointment system to cope with the needs of the elderly. Sensible repeat prescription scheme, with 'fail safe' device for regular checks. Suitable surveillance for wanted and unwanted effects What will happen when they have minor illness?

12. What about the carers? Day to day assistance from home help, nurse, meals on wheels, local voluntary groups?
Holiday admissions?
Regular contacts and counselling with doctor, health visitor, nurse, social worker?
Day centres/units?
Nursing homes – how to arrange finance?

Challenges

○ Do I know who my over-75s are?
○ Do I know their problems and needs?
○ How to cope with likely increasing work load?
○ How best to use available people and resources?

Suggestions

○ Age/sex register to identify the elderly
○ Assess routine care of the aged. Delegate follow-up work where possible and concentrate as GP on medical work
○ Consider simple screening perhaps yearly, but concentrate on any danger periods, e.g. after discharge from hospital, or after death of spouse
○ Find out what facilities there are to help old people in the area and what are the gaps
○ Help to get the gaps filled – after all: 'where they tread, we follow'.

A7 Terminal Care

Objectives

1. Terminal care means looking after any patient in the last weeks of life. It is not restricted to death from painful malignancy.

2. The patient should *'die well'* and with dignity. He needs a physician who will help him throughout the illness, and not retreat into professionalism.

3. It presumes total patient care in the patient's preferred context – home, hospice or hospital.

Problems

○ **The right setting.** About one third of deaths in the UK occur at home. The patient may want to die at home but may not be able to do so because of lack of nursing or medical support, or because his family are not prepared to cope. Changing this may mean vigorous campaigning for nursing and family support.

○ **Common symptoms.** In order of frequency

- pain
- poor sleep
- loss of appetite
- constipation/diarrhoea
- nausea/vomiting
- incontinence – faecal/urinary
- cough
- breathlessness
- depression/anxiety
- confusion
- bad smells
- bed sores
- pruritus

Towards end of life majority become physically restricted and some (1 in 5) completely bedbound.

○ **Pain control.** Little or no pain may be experienced by some of patients dying from cancer: but of the remainder, one half experience severe pain. Many are given too little analgesia too late. There is much fear in the community of cancer and death. As a result pain is made worse by fear, loneliness, depression, anxiety, hypercalcaemia, infection and anticipation of pain to come. Acute pain is an event with a meaning: chronic pain is an endless situation devoid of satisfactory explanation for the patient, frequently expanding to fill all his conscious self and isolating him from the world around him.

○ **Isolation.** Many of the dying are physically and emotionally alone, surrounded by a conspiracy of silence, with visitors driven away by fear, embarrassment or distaste. Neither medical staff nor relatives may welcome discussion. The precise understanding of diagnosis and prognosis, however, may be much less important for the patient than the knowledge that someone cares and is ready to share some of his concerns.

○ Stages of acceptance of diagnosis and prognosis.
These are well recognized, although not always passed through or needed.

1. The patient may begin by **denying** the diagnosis, either verbally or in behaviour, in spite of explanation. The patient may show ambivalence and may press the doctor to offer alternative explanations or further referrals.

2. This may be replaced by **anger or blame** – *'why me?'* – *'why was it not detected before?'* No one can do the right thing, and if doctor and relatives are not prepared to cope with their guilt the patient may be deserted.

3. Some patients **bargain** by offering alternative ways of proceeding, to *'buy off'* the disease.

4. Most patients go through a stage of **depression** when it is clear that they cannot avoid the truth any longer. This may be masked by a superficial cheerfulness: it may be short, or it may merge with the mood and level of consciousness of the last days. If it is persistent and severe it may be helped by antidepressant treatment, but often careful and open handling and discussion when the patient indicates that the time is ripe will lead to –

5. **Acceptance.** Enough time and help is needed to work through the previous stages. It may not be a state of obvious happiness, but one where the patient sleeps a lot, and may finally slip into the quietness that surrounds his last hours.

○ **Relatives need support** – perhaps more than the patient – especially if they cannot cope with a discussion of the true diagnosis. It is the patient's illness, but they must be prepared for their loss.

○ **Our own fears.** Most studies show that doctors and nurses for the most part are more afraid of death, and of speaking about it, than their dying patients. Some think that the patient who asks no questions is protecting his medical attendants from a task he knows they do not relish. *'What do you let your patients tell you?'*

○ **Speaking to the dying**
Doctors are not good at talking to the dying. This may be because we feel helpless, or that we have failed. We may not be reconciled to our own death.

The patient will usually indicate when he wants us to talk, and he should not be rushed. An open question *'Perhaps you are wondering how bad this illness is?'* may be a cue that is taken up, or left.

Some may never want to know and we should not press them. Direct questions from the patient should get direct but supportive encouraging answers. The patient may start by telling us what *he* knows. Often the questions will be *'Will it be painful?' 'How long have I got?'* Unexpected fears may be uncovered, of what it will be like at the end, about who will look after family or pets. Sometimes it may be important to ask if the patient is afraid of dying, and why, so that we can reassure them that we will support them all through. Sometimes it may be important just to sit together in calm silence.

Organization	GP	○ 24 hour cover
		○ plan of care and institutional back-up
		○ knowledge or access to knowledge of plan by colleagues
		○ access to relevant drugs
		○ allocation of key worker, not necessarily GP, who will have main relationship with patient and relatives
		○ procedure at the death and patient's or relative's wishes
		○ personal visit to relatives after death
	District Nurse	○ fully involved even if not attached to practice
	Health Visitor	○ especially for children and elderly

Hospital or Hospice team may be available to visit at home and prepare for the final inpatient stay if required.

Admission to hospital or hospice should not be delayed if home care becomes difficult. Where possible this should be preceded by a home visit from hospice or domiciliary visit by consultant.

Pain control

General principles

1. Analgesics must be given regularly **prophylactically** before pain recurs (3–4 hourly for opiates).

2. Use **oral** therapy for as long as possible. Suppositories may be an alternative. Injections can usually be reserved for last days or even hours.

3. Dosage should rapidly be increased to control pain completely: then can sometimes be diminished gradually when control established.

4. All other symptoms (e.g. itch, sleeplessness, loneliness, depression) may worsen pain perception and must also be tackled.

5. Neither physical dependence nor tolerance need be practical problems if opiates are given within a programme of total care.

Analgesics

Have a '**League Table**' of analgesics:

MINOR   *viz* aspirin ⟶ indomethacin (bone and joint pain)
or paracetamol ⟶ Co-proxanol or dihydrocodeine (other pain)

MEDIUM   *viz* dipipanone (Diconal)
or dextromoramide (Palfium) and suppositories

STRONG   morphine or diamorphine

Remember **alternative forms** of pain relief – e.g. radiotherapy, cytotoxics, nerve blocks.

Consider **hypercalcaemia,** which can precipitate or exacerbate pain; if present, can be treated with steroids.

Use **laxative** with opiates, as well as antiemetic (e.g. metoclopramide or cyclizine).

Other symptoms	**Breathlessness**

Breathlessness
○ Non-specific
  – prednisolone initially 20–30 mg, reducing as necessary, to reduce wheezing and tumour mass.
  – low-dose opiates to control tachypnoea and allay anxiety
  – theophylline derivatives (long acting)
  – salbutamol or other bronchodilators

○ Specific
  – diuretics
  – digoxin
  – oxygen
  – antibiotics, for infections
  – pleural effusion tap
  – radiotherapy and/or chemotherapy

Cough
○ Physiotherapy for expectoration and drainage
○ Antibiotics
○ Cough suppressants
  – codeine/pholcodeine linctus
  – methadone linctus
  – diamorphine linctus
  – prednisolone
○ Nebulizer
  – sterile water humidification
  – bupivacaine/salbutamol etc

Poor appetite
○ Correct correctable causes
○ Prednisolone
○ Appetizers, such as alcohol, if desired, or others

Vomiting
○ Check for side effects of drugs such as opiates
○ Check for faecal impaction or hypercalcaemia
○ Antiemetics
  – metoclopramide
  – prochloperazine
  – cyclizine
  – chlorpromazine
○ dexamethasone – high doses (2–8 mg) reducing

Pruritus
Possible causes jaundice, allergies, melanomatosis.
○ Trimeprazine
○ Steroids – prednisolone or methylprednisolone
○ Cholestyramine or methyltestosterone in jaundice

Sore dry mouth
Frequent in terminally ill, candidosis often the cause.
○ Nystatin oral suspension
○ Oral toilets
○ Fluids ++

Bed sores, incontinence, colostomies, wounds
○ All need skilled frequent nursing care
○ Try and minimize bad smells
○ Remember incontinent laundry services

Constipation
Frequent ++, unpleasant and often missed. Empty rectum does not exclude.
○ Evacuate lower bowel and rectum with enemas, suppositories or manual evacuation (under analgesia)
○ Roughage diet or bulk producing substances
○ Regular laxatives
  - danthron
  - lactulose
  - senna products
  - biscodyl

Hiccoughs
○ Chlorpromazine
○ Perphenazine
○ Metoclopramide
○ Haloperidol
○ Hyoscine

Depression
Understandably reactive, fear, sadness and misery are frequent. Drugs play small part. Good human care is best.

Possibly use tricyclic or tetracyclic antidepressives in some cases.
○ amitriptyline
○ mianserin

Poor sleep
Hypnotics should only be used after pain and other symptoms have been treated.
○ Try night cap of alcohol
○ Short acting benzodiazepines
○ Phenothiazines for the agitated

Bereavement
Grief takes many forms
○ Shock and denial may be first reactions
○ Guilt may follow as realities sink in
○ Blame of self, doctors, nurses and others available
○ Anger against deceased, mourners, clergy and even God
○ Relief, often with uncertainty and unease
○ New and recurring illness and symptoms in bereaved
○ Hallucinations about continuing presence of dead person may lead to thoughts of insanity
○ Severe psychiatric reactions, i.e. depression, fugues or even suicide

Bereaved must be given opportunities to talk, to be comforted and reassured that she/he did all possible for deceased and that death was a 'happy release' and continuing life would have meant continuing suffering.

A8   Care of Immigrants

Whilst immigrant patients in general require the same kind of care as any other group, they do have some special difficulties and problems which the doctor should be aware of.

Language

Whilst some immigrant groups speak English as their native language, others have no knowledge of the language so the doctor will need the services of an appropriate interpreter. Possible sources are members of the patient's family or the doctor's employed or attached staff. In case of difficulty the local Community Relations Council may be able to help. The Health Education Council provides leaflets on a wide variety of topics in Hindi, Urdu, Punjabi and Gujerati.

Culture

The variety of cultural differences in and between the various immigrant groups and the native population are so great that it is quite impossible to summarize them here. The general practitioner should try to become familiar with the cultural norms of his own local immigrant population. Some of the main areas in which difficulties may arise are listed below.

Names

This can be a particular problem with Asian immigrants from the Indian subcontinent or East Africa. It is important to encourage a systematic approach by the staff in recording Asian names and to encourage the patients to bring their NHS medical cards with them to the surgery. An up-to-date street index, with the names grouped according to the individual houses in which patients live, can be extremely helpful, especially for home visits.

Family structure and housing

Whilst many West Indian children are brought up in single-parent families, Asian children are very likely to be part of a large extended family network. However, this system too has its problems in that the daughter-in-law in effect marries the whole of her husband's extended family and often comes to live with them. Since most houses in Britain are small and designed for nuclear families these often become overcrowded. Paradoxically, this may lead to isolation and unhappiness, especially if she is tied at home with young children whilst her husband works long hours away from home. Nevertheless, the nursing of sick members of the family and the care of the elderly are greatly facilitated within the extended family system.

Illness behaviour

Patients coming from Africa or Asia often have very different experience of the significance of symptoms to that of the British doctor. A child with a fever in some parts of the world is quite likely to be developing a serious or even fatal illness and thus the parents may overreact by our standards. Thus there may be inappropriate requests for home visits or out-of-hours calls which can cause irritation. Similarly, catarrhal symptoms in both children and adults are much more common in the UK and often lead to multiple consultations for symptomatic relief. Few immigrant patients are likely to present to their doctors complaining of depression or unhappiness, instead the symptoms are somatized to headaches, backaches or even 'whole-body pain'. Traditional healers from their own background are available in most immigrant communities and may well be more helpful in these situations because of their knowledge of the patient's cultural background.

Muslim women, in particular, are often reluctant to be examined by a male doctor, and this may cause problems in obstetrics, gynaecology and family planning. The attitude of the husband is often a crucial factor.

Experience suggests that the illness behaviour of immigrant patients tends to become similar to that of the natives over the period of a few years, whilst the immigrants' children adopt most of the cultural norms of their adopted society.

Medical problems

Calcium + vitamin D deficiency (in Asians): neonatal convulsions, rickets, osteomalacia.
○ Caused by insufficient dietary intake, restricted exposure to u.v. light.
○ Can be prevented and treated by vitamin D + calcium supplements (BNF).

Tuberculosis (particularly in Asian patients): may affect cervical lymph nodes, lungs, bones, GU tract or CNS.
○ May be detected early by routine chest X-ray of all new Asian patients and a high index of suspicion.
○ May be reduced in incidence by good nutrition and housing plus the administration of BCG vaccine to all babies born into Asian immigrant households and to tuberculin-negative child contacts of infectious patients.
○ Treatment is routine and highly effective.

Malaria (in any patient coming from the tropics): often presents as a non-specific pyrexial illness.
○ Should be considered in any pyrexial patient returning from a malarial zone. When in doubt, take a specimen of blood in an ordinary sequestrene bottle and send to Lab.
○ Can be prevented by adequate chemoprophylaxis and treated relatively easily once diagnosed (BNF).

Anaemia (especially in young children and strictly vegetarian Hindu women): often presents as non-specific weakness or tiredness.
○ Easily detected if high index of suspicion.
○ Iron deficiency is most common but patients may also be deficient in B_{12} and folate.
○ May be prevented and treated by more liberal diet, supplemented as necessary by oral iron, vitamin B_{12} and folic acid (BNF).

Sickle-cell trait (occurs in 10% of negroid immigrants): may present with recurrent pain in the abdomen and legs ± jaundice, ocular symptoms, haematuria and anaemia (sickle-cell disease).
○ May be detected by a positive sickling test and electrophoresis.
○ May be prevented by screening all negro patients before administering a general anaesthetic, flying or other exposure to hypoxic conditions.

Thalassaemia (especially in Mediterranean immigrants): (1) anaemia, massive splenomegaly, stunting of growth and development (*thalassaemia major*); (2) mild anaemia, aggravated by pregnancy (*thalassaemia minor*).
○ May be confirmed by haemoglobin electrophoresis – increased HbA_2 + fetal Hb.
○ The anaemia is unresponsive to iron but may be improved by folic acid therapy.

Intestinal parasites (in patients from the tropics): often asymptomatic.
○ Stool examination should be considered early in any patient with diarrhoea, abdominal pain or general malaise.
○ Treatment is usually simple (BNF)

Peptic ulcers (especially in Asian immigrants)
○ High incidence is presumably related to dietary habits.
○ Treatment is routine, but particular attention should be paid to dietary factors.

Mental illness
○ Incidence of psychotic illness is probably similar to native population, but is often more difficult to detect and comprehend.
○ Neurotic symptoms are more likely to be somatized.
○ Prevention and treatment are much more difficult if the members of the primary health care team are not familiar with the patient's cultural and social background.

A9   Care of the Disabled

Scope and opportunity

○ The majority of disabled people on any general practitioner's list could be identified within a year.
○ Planned care could reduce the amount of misery and degree of disability of the disabled.
○ Support, relief and provision of aids could extend the time a disabled person can remain in the community.
○ Early recognition and appropriate action could prevent breakdown in caring relatives and enable them to carry on longer.

Objectives

1. To facilitate as high a quality of life as possible in all respects.

2. To preserve independence and self-confidence.

3. To limit increasing disability and restrict its effects (tertiary prevention).

4. To recognize and treat intercurrent illness at an early stage.

5. To recognize need for help, know of what help is available and make sure the need is met as far as it can be.

6. To be aware of the effects of the individual's disability on relatives and provide support and relief where possible.

Problems

1. The disabled, like the elderly, **often fail to seek help**, partly because they do not know what is available and partly because they want to appear to be independent and coping well. Some are also afraid that if they admit to difficulties they will be 'put away'.

2. **Psychological problems** are common. Soon after a disability develops, if it has not been present from early life, there is a reaction, a bit like bereavement. The patient may be shocked, denying, angry, resentful, blaming and depressed in turn or all at once. Help may be needed over a long period if the individual is to get through this period with a minimum of permanent damage and start to make the most of what he can do. Thereafter there is always the risk of depression particularly if the degree of dependence is high or increasing. Everyone needs to be needed.

3. **Domestic organization** can be improved by the provision of appropriate aids. Someone in the primary health care team should have a knowledge of what is available and how it can be obtained. (*See list* at end of section.) A Home Help may be needed but sometimes only occasionally or when there is another problem, e.g. intercurrent illness or absence of helpful neighbour or caring relative.

   Housing may have to be specially built or adapted.

4. **Social life, work, occupation** are vital. Boredom and isolation can have serious effects: lethargy, inertia, decreasing alertness, withdrawal and depression. Activity reduces the likelihood of physical results of inertia, such as pressure sores, contractures and D.V.T. Sport for the disabled is available in many areas and includes riding, swimming and wheelchair sports such as table tennis, archery and weight training. Yoga is

particularly helpful for disabled people. Clubs in most areas cater for the disabled.

Sheltered workshops, day centres and occupational therapy at home or in a centre may be available.

5. **Mobility** should be maintained as far as possible. Aids of increasing sophistication are becoming available – some from the DHSS, some only privately. Funds may be available from injury compensation or from charitable funds. There is an artificial limb and appliance centre (ALAC) for every area.

6. **Families** can often care for the most profoundly disabled people for long periods if they have support and intermittent relief. Day care, evening sitters, weekend and holiday admissions to hospital or special units all help.

7. **Liaison with other agencies** such as social workers, WRVS and other charitable organizations is essential.

8. **Finance**
Most disabled people suffer financial hardship.

Their earning capacity is less and their needs greater than other people.

They are less able to economize and make do.

They have to pay for repairs and maintenance which fit people might carry out themselves.

Allowances are minimal but it is important that they know about and claim all they are entitled to. Social worker, health visitor and DHSS should all be able to advise about this.

Statistics

10% of the population under 65 years are disabled.

90% of the disabled see their general practitioner in any year.

10% never see any other professional.

50% of the difficulties of daily living reported by the disabled may be unknown to their GPs.

Allowances

Non-contributory invalidity pension
For people of working age who can't get sickness benefit but who have not been able to work for at least 28 weeks. Married women can qualify if they are also unable to do normal household duties.

Supplementary benefit
'The difference between what you need each week and the money you have coming in each week.' Other payments under this heading are allowances for extra heating, laundry, domestic help, diet and other unspecified 'special expenses'. It is not payable to people with savings more than a set amount nor to those whose income is above the base level in operation at the time. Certain items of income are excluded from the calculations, including the attendance and mobility allowances.

Attendance allowance
You must be so severely disabled that for 6 months you have needed:

By day

○ frequent attention throughout the day in connection with your bodily functions, or

○ continual supervision throughout the day in order to avoid substantial danger to yourself or others.

or

By night

○ prolonged or repeated attention during the night in connection with your bodily functions, or

○ continual supervision throughout the night in order to avoid substantial danger to yourself or others.

The claim is decided on medical grounds.

Mobility allowance
Can be claimed by people between 5 and 65 who are unable, or almost unable, to walk because of physical disablement. If entitlement is established before the 66th birthday, the allowance may be continued until the age of 75. The allowance is made on medical grounds only, regardless of financial circumstances, but it is subject to income tax.

Free prescriptions
Are available to anyone receiving supplementary benefit or family income supplement.

Hospital patient's travelling expenses
Are payable to anyone receiving supplementary benefit or family income supplement.

Exemption from road tax and exemption from rates on a garage
May be given to people receiving mobility allowance and to some others.

Assistance with fares to work
Is available to some disabled people.

Invalid care allowance
Is payable to men and single women of working age who are unable to work because they have to stay at home to look after a severely disabled relative who is getting attendance allowance.

Industrial injury benefit, industrial disablement benefit, industrial death benefit and special benefits for industrial diseases such as pneumoconiosis are payable in certain circumstances.

Rent and rate rebates are payable to some people on low incomes who do not receive supplementary benefit.

People with massive lump sum compensation may need professional financial advice and protection from exploitation.

Special terms for buying a car and other goods and services
Arranged by the Royal Association for Disability and Rehabilitation, 23/25 Mortimer Street, London, W1N 8AB.

The Family Fund, Joseph Rowntree Memorial Trust, Beverly House, Skipton Lane, York Y03 6RB provides financial and other help for families with severely handicapped children under 16.

Leaflet HB:1 '**Help for handicapped people**' from DHSS is very useful as are several others from the same source.

(**Also consider** suggestions listed in A.6, Care of the Elderly.)

Organization

○ It is important to try to identify problems before they become crises. It may help to keep some sort of register or card index of disabled people to facilitate regular review.

○ One member of the primary health care team could act as Keyworker for each disabled person. Who takes on this role depends on the problems the patient has, i.e. who is already involved, and the availability of staff. This individual could liaise with other agencies, e.g. chiropody, physio, DHSS, WRVS.

Section B

TEACHING AND LEARNING

B1 Patient Education

The Need

○ A vast amount of disease and disability is self-inflicted by unhealthy lifestyle, dangerous practices or neglect of sensible safety precautions.
○ Many families are ignorant of how to manage minor illness, or how to work with professionals in the management of more complex conditions.
○ There is widespread ignorance of what services are available and how they should be used.

Whose Job is it?

○ The primary health care team is not the only source of information but it is an important one.
○ Others are
  − the media: radio, TV, newspapers, magazines
  − schools with or without help from health professionals
  − District Health Authorities; Health Education − local clinics
  − hospitals, e.g. in antenatal clinics

How is it done?

Patient education occurs at a number of different levels and in different ways.

Every contact with the practice by telephone, letter or in person has some educational content even though neither party may be aware of it at the time.

It is important that this content is as deliberate and beneficial as possible. To be effective, all teaching has to be consistent and oft repeated.

Content

The aim is that everyone should know how to live a healthy life, manage minor ailments and make proper use of the services.

Healthy life-style

○ **Diet** should be eaten as regular meals and should contain:

  ○ more fruit, vegetables, fish, roughage
  ○ less animal fats, sugar, salt
  ○ sufficient to maintain optimum weight
  ○ help may be needed by the obese to lose weight.

○ **Smoking:** Everyone should be encouraged to stop or at least cut down, especially those with other risk factors.

The dangers should be known to all.

○ **Alcohol** should be taken in moderation or not at all, minimally in pregnancy
  - Everyone needs to know the risks and warning signs of excessive drinking.
  - These are played down by society as a whole and not least by doctors themselves, who have a high incidence of alcoholism and alcohol-related diseases.
  - It may be helpful in small quantities as an analgesic, cough suppressant, sedative and hypnotic.
  - All heavy drinkers are at serious risk and many would not consider themselves heavy drinkers.
  - A heavy drinker is a man who drinks more than 50 units a week or a woman who drinks more than 25 units a week.
  - A unit is a $\frac{1}{2}$ pint of beer, pub single of spirits, small sherry, or 1 glass of wine.
  - Any man who averages $3\frac{1}{2}$ pints of beer a day or a woman who has a small sherry, $1\frac{1}{2}$ glasses of wine and a small whisky every evening, is a heavy drinker.
  - This level of intake over a long period damages many organs but especially brain and liver, which are most sensitive.
  - Any alcohol at all affects driving ability: it is not enough to be within the legal limit.
  - No one should take any alcohol within 48 hours of a dose of tranquillizer or hypnotic.

○ Drugs

Prescribed drugs such as tranquillizers have the most widespread effect. Hypnotics may be addictive after 3 consecutive days' use.

Tranquillizers are mostly prescribed for women and are very difficult to stop once tolerance has developed. Withdrawal effects can be severe and the dose has to be reduced over a long period. During this time the patient may need regular support from GP, Health Visitor or community psychiatric nurse.

Benzodiazepines should only be prescribed for patients suffering from severe psychiatric illness.

They have no place in the management of normal people suffering from life crises or stressful situations.

Cannabis (hashish, marijuana) has not been proven to have any long term serious harmful physical effects, except that the smoke has a high tar content and since it is usually smoked with tobacco, has all the dangers of cigarette smoking.

Opiates (morphine, heroin, methadone). The amount of illegal opiates being used is increasing worldwide.

Not all users are addicts.

Heroin may be injected, or sniffed, or heated and inhaled ('chasing the dragon').

It is more dangerous when injected because of the risks of septicaemia, hepatitis and overdose.

It is equally addictive whichever route is chosen and most addicts end up injecting.

Heroin is often used with other drugs such as cocaine.

Some drug users take or inject a great variety of drugs, including amphetamines, barbiturates and benzodiazepines. The barbiturates are the most dangerous.

Injection of and addiction to barbiturates is more dangerous than to heroin.

Dangers of heroin addiction: Under controlled conditions of dosage and administration, heroin causes no physical harm.
- The risks arise from malnutrition (because the cost of the drug and the lifestyle often leave little time, money or appetite for food); septicaemia and hepatitis B; social isolation and deterioration.
- A heroin addict has a 2½-fold risk of death compared with someone else of the same age.
- Ten years after the beginning of addiction, about half the addicts are fit and well and off the drug. This number is not influenced by medical treatment, nor is the number of deaths.
- Most heroin addicts are unknown to their GPs.
- The GP's role is to comfort and support the family and to be available if ever the addict himself needs someone to turn to or develops complications which need treatment.

Methadone is prescribed to 80% of notified addicts. It is supposed to be taken orally but is often injected. It seems to be more difficult to stop than heroin.

There is much debate about its use.

Solvent abuse – See under Section A.4, 'The Adolescent', page 64.

○ **Exercise** should be regular and comfortably strenuous. Men over 40 should be warned not to play squash or other intensely strenuous competitive games.

○ **Stress** is unavoidable and a necessary stimulus. Everyone needs to recognize when it is excessive or when someone is failing to cope with it: then what to do about it.

○ **Accidents:** Children and the elderly are particularly vulnerable.

1. *At home*: Fire guards, cooker rails, flame resistant clothing, stair gates, storage for medicines and dangerous chemicals, harnesses for pram and high chairs, and most of all a watchful parent.

2. *On roads*: Never drink and drive (any alcohol makes driving dangerous: not just the legal limit); never allow young children out alone, never sit child on lap of front seat passenger. Always use seat belts, including rear ones; teach children crossing drill.

Management of illness

Many people are ignorant of the normal bodily functions and need information about growth, sleep requirements, bowel function, menstruation, appetite, micturition and sexual function. Everyone also needs to be able to recognize serious symptoms such as chest pain or rectal bleeding.

○ **Self-care**. Except in the very young, frail or elderly, self-care should be possible in:
Short-lived fevers (less than 2–3 days) without other symptoms.
Epidemic diarrhoea and vomiting without pain or blood.
Mild indigestion and hangovers.

Upper respiratory tract infections.

Muscular strains and bruises, insect bites, grazes.

Headache which is not severe, prolonged or accompanied by vomiting.

Backache which is not severe, prolonged or accompanied by difficulty in micturition.

Rashes if patient is otherwise well and not taking medicines.

○ **Assisted self-care**. In a further number of situations, self-care is combined with treatment or advice from a member of the primary health care team. These include

Acute conditions such as otitis media or heart failure when drugs are prescribed;

Chronic conditions such as diabetes, hypertension or asthma.

The outcome in all these situations depends on the intelligent application of general measures such as bed rest, diet and over-the-counter medicines (such as aspirin and paracetamol) and on the ability to co-operate in treatment regimens prescribed by the doctor (q.v.).

Use of services

Primary Health Care Team: The patients need to know who the personnel are, what they do and when and how to seek their advice. A 'rogue's gallery' of photographs and labels is helpful and can be posted up in a prominent place near the reception desk or in the waiting room.

Other agencies: Information is also needed about what is available and when and how to use all the following:
1. Hospital – especially A. & E. department and walk-in clinics like VD and alcoholics.
2. Child Guidance Clinic
3. Social Services Department
4. Police – especially Juvenile Bureau
5. Probation Service
6. Lawyers; legal aid service and free advice session
7. Family Planning Clinic
8. Voluntary Agencies
    - Citizens Advice Bureau
    - WRVS
    - Marriage Guidance Council
    - Samaritans
    - Churches
    - NSPCC
    - Care Groups
    - Special Groups, e.g. M.S. Society, British Diabetic Association, Alcoholics groups

Methods

○ **Personal (verbal) information** is probably the most valuable, especially that given by the GP directly to the patient.

However, it is often misunderstood or forgotten and needs reinforcement.

One way of doing this is by supplying written advice. This can be handwritten at the time – very effective, if legible, but time consuming – or in the form of a standard leaflet.

Another very effective form of reinforcement is by a follow-up visit by a nurse or health visitor.

○ **Patient advice leaflets**. Can apply to anything from how to manage a cold or take a drug to how to lose weight or use a contraceptive.
   - Many are produced by pharmaceutical companies and inform about particular conditions or drugs.
   - Those written by the practice for their own use are more likely to coincide with the verbal advice being given.
   - They can be freely available to anyone who wants them or can be given to patients individually to reinforce verbal advice.
   - Some are produced in languages other than English.

○ **Practice information booklets** range from a single card with doctors' names, surgery hours and telephone numbers, to a complete health care manual including everything in this section.

○ **Also consider the following**:
   Posters
   Tape-slide presentations
   Small groups to look at particular issues like child care or problems of the disabled
   Small groups of overweight people to diet and exercise
   Groups with back problems to do exercises
   Many excellent leaflets are available from the Health Education Council at 78 New Oxford Street, London, WC1

Undergraduate Education

The attitudes of both medical schools and medical students to general practice have changed in the last twenty years, and now there is much interest in the community as an area where students should have some of their training. Much is owed to the Todd Report, changes in curriculum and exams to include GP studies, and the foundation of new universities where behavioural studies feature largely in the curriculum. The cynical might also claim that the improved financial status of the GP and his relative freedom from bureaucratic restrictions in comparison with his hospital colleagues have added to students' interest. However, when a student visits a practice, both student and GP can be seen to benefit and it is hoped more practitioners will feel able to take part in undergraduate education at all levels. If you feel that you might be interested in teaching medical students, contact the Department of General Practice in your Regional Medical School for further information.

The schemes

There are **two types** of scheme:

1. The **newer medical courses** have community or human development studies which are taught from the beginning of training, and much of this teaching draws resources from general practice. A student may:

   (a) meet a patient in his own home and see his problem there in context;

   (b) follow a normal human process through its various stages – such as following a mother through her pregnancy and delivery and visiting her and the child in subsequent years;

   (c) help as an unqualified worker in old people's clubs or day centres, or act as co-therapist in psychotherapeutic exercises;

   (d) visit practices to understand how community services are organized;

   (e) visit practices to sit in with the doctor and see patients.

2. The **older medical courses** have revised their curricula to fit general practice into a conventional timetable of 'firm' attachments, either as a residential block, or by day-release during another 'firm' like psychiatry. Here a proportion of the week is spent with a GP in practice and the students come back to the medical school for regular seminar or group teaching. Some schools use both methods combined with some teaching by GPs joining the normal ward programme.

   Some schools have full time academic staff but many do not and depend on sessional teachers also acting as general practitioners. Funding restrictions usually do not allow more than a nominal remuneration to GPs taking students, together with reimbursement of residential expenses, but it is hoped that this situation will be improved in the future. If you are taking a student into your practice, it is very important to read letters of instruction from the academic staff carefully and keep them for reference.

The aims of these schemes

1. To introduce students to the 85% of illness episodes which do not need hospital care, and the different spectrum of illness and style of presentation in practice.

2. To show students how normal men and women, of different classes and backgrounds from their own, live and work.

3. To demonstrate 'whole person' diagnosis, and how social and family pressures impinge on health.

4. To watch and take part in the general practice consultation.

5. To meet other community health workers, whether employed by local authority or attached to a practice, and to understand their roles and how they work.

Side effects

Often students have not followed a doctor through his whole working day, and may never have had a one-to-one relationship with a qualified doctor. They may never have considered working in the community, or may have a distorted view of practice from their experiences in hospital. 'To be actually getting down to it' and doing essential medical work may be very exciting, and the GP should give the student any work with patients that the student is keen and able to do.

Methods

1. **Sitting in with the GP**
   The student should always be introduced to the patient and the patient's permission for his presence obtained. Show the student the different style of consultation from the hospital, with a series of short consultations, often involving no examination or special tests, on patients about whom data is gradually collected;
   - general practice records;
   - 'games' in the surgery, body language, 'while I'm here', 'it's me again, doc';
   - the unexpected or absent patient, e.g. the depressed mother presenting via her child, the wife discussing her alcoholic husband;
   - the wide variation of presenting problems including many not strictly medical: 'ticket of entry'.
   - the multitude of symptomatology, the need to explain what patients have not got, how to sift major from minor problems;
   - prescribing.
   Most doctors find that the extra time taken up with the student is more than compensated for by the happy way in which these sessions are received by the patients. However, a strategy should be organized for the student when it is clear his presence is inhibitory. Some doctors have given experienced students the doctor's chair while sitting by him, or have asked their patients to see the student initially before consulting the doctor, and then discussed the problem together. Final year medical students may well be able to manage patients to a large extent, with supervision.

2. **Introduction**
   Lay aside time at the beginning to introduce the student to all the staff, and to your family if appropriate. Learn about what he has done so far, his interests and ambitions, the gaps in his knowledge, and what you can learn from him. He may be a pharmacologist, sailing half-blue or jazz fiend.

3. **Meeting the practice team**
   Suggestions include sitting in the waiting room, with the receptionists, with the health visitor, district or practice nurses, joining baby clinics. Include the student in all discussions and conferences where possible and appropriate.

4. **Visiting**
   Do not shield him from any valuable experiences and let him visit with the health visitor or nurse too. Consider asking him to get to know one family or problem in some depth over his time with you, perhaps writing up a project on a patient with a chronic illness, a dying patient, or a handicapped patient and family.

5. **The community**
   Arrange for him to visit any organization or centre locally you think is valuable, such as a day centre, prison, chemist, mental handicap group, or any facility that the area has. Make sure he sees what the area can offer for social life and leisure too.

6. **Projects and evaluation**
   The medical school may have set him a project – if so, help him with material for it.
   The school may require an evaluation of the student. If they permit, discuss it with him before he leaves. You may be the first to point out to him that he bites his nails in consultations, that he should be a paediatrician or that no one can read his writing. Praise as well as criticize. You need never see him again: but if you would like to, suggest another meeting.

B3 Vocational Training

The following job description for the general practitioner and educational aims for vocational training were set out by a working party appointed by the Second European Conference on the teaching of general practice. They were subsequently adopted by the Joint Committee on Postgraduate Training for General Practice (JCPTGP), the Royal College of General Practitioners and the Council for Postgraduate Medical Education in England and Wales.

Description of work

The general practitioner is a licensed medical graduate who gives personal, primary and continuing care to individuals, families and a practice population, irrespective of age, sex and illness. It is the synthesis of these functions which is unique. He will attend his patients in his consulting room and in their homes and sometimes in a clinic or a hospital. His aim is to make early diagnoses. He will include and integrate physical, psychological and social factors in his considerations about health and illness. This will be expressed in the care of his patients. He will make an initial decision about every problem which is presented to him as a doctor. He will undertake the continuing management of his patients with chronic, recurrent or terminal illnesses. Prolonged contact means that he can use repeated opportunities to gather information at a pace appropriate to each patient and build up a relationship of trust which he can use professionally. He will practise in co-operation with other colleagues, medical and non-medical. He will know how and when to intervene through treatment, prevention and education to promote the health of his patients and their families. He will recognize that he also has a professional responsibility to the community.

Educational aims

At the conclusion of the training programme the doctor should be able to demonstrate:

1. **Knowledge**
   (a)   that he has sufficient knowledge of disease processes, particularly of common diseases, chronic diseases and those which endanger life or have serious complications or consequences.
   (b)   that he understands the opportunities, methods and limitations of prevention, early diagnoses and management in the setting of general practice.
   (c)   his understanding of the way in which interpersonal relationships within the family can cause health problems or alter their presentation, course and management, just as illness can influence family relationships.
   (d)   an understanding of the social and environmental circumstances of his patients and how they may affect a relationship between health and illness.
   (e)   his knowledge and appropriate use of the wide range of interventions available to him.
   (f)   that he understands the ethics of his profession and their importance for the patient.
   (g)   that he understands the basic methods of research as applied to general practice.

(h)   an understanding of medico-social legislation and of the impact of this on his patient.

2.   Skills

(a)   how to form diagnoses which take account of physical, psychological and social factors.

(b)   that he understands the use of epidemiology and probability in his everyday work.

(c)   understanding the use of the factor (time) as a diagnostic, therapeutic and organizational tool.

(d)   that he can identify persons at risk and take appropriate action.

(e)   that he can make relevant initial decisions about every problem presented to him as a doctor.

(f)   the capacity to co-operate with medical and non-medical professionals.

(g)   knowledge and appropriate use of the skills of practice management.

3.   Attitudes

(a)   a capacity for empathy and for forming a specific and effective relationship with patients and for developing a degree of self-understanding.

(b)   how his recognition of the patient as a unique individual modifies the way in which he elicits information and makes hypotheses about the nature of his problems and their management.

(c)   that he understands that helping patients to solve their own problems is a fundamental therapeutic activity.

(d)   that he recognizes that he can make a professional contribution to the wider community.

(e)   that he is willing and able critically to evaluate his own work.

(f)   that he recognizes his own need for continuing education and critical reading of medical information.

Vocational Training Regulations

Since August 1982 all doctors wishing to be appointed as a principal in general medical practice in the NHS must have completed a course of prescribed or equivalent experience, approved by the Joint Committee on Postgraduate Training for General Practice (JCPTGP).

Prescribed experience implies a minimum of 3 years full time post-registration training, including 1 year as a trainee in an approved teaching practice and 2 years in educationally approved posts in hospital. The hospital component of training must include at least 6 months in any two of the following relevant specialities.

General Medicine
Geriatrics
Accident and Emergency (or General Surgery)
Psychiatry
Paediatrics
Obstetrics and/or Gynaecology

The other hospital year may include posts of any duration in any specialty provided that they are educationally approved by the appropriate Royal College.

Those doctors who do not fulfil the criteria for prescribed experience may apply to the JCPT, with details of their curriculum vitae, if they consider that their experience may be equivalent to that prescribed by the regulations. The JCPTGP, 14 Princes Gate, London, SW7 1PU will then give guidance if any further training is required in order to satisfy the regulations.

During the year in general practice all trainees are expected to attend Trainer–Trainee Meetings and day or half-day release courses. In some Vocational Training Schemes the associated academic course extends throughout the 3 years.

The present situation is that there are places available for about 50% of all GP trainees on organized 3-year schemes which provide a 'package' of hospital and general practice training posts recognized as suitable pre-scribed experience by the JCPTGP. The other 50% of trainees need to construct a suitable programme of training for themselves and are advised to seek the advice of their Regional Adviser in General Practice at an early stage in case of doubt or difficulty about appropriate posts.

Group Activities for Trainee GPs

There are two types of group learning situations available for trainees.

Trainer/trainee groups usually meet locally, often over lunch, for $1-1\frac{1}{2}$ hours, and provide an informal opportunity for all the trainers and trainees in a district to meet and get to know each other, exchange ideas, discuss topics of general interest to GPs and identify those areas where outside expertise may be valuable.

Day or half-day release courses are organized on a district or subregional basis depending on requirements. Normally the course organizer will be the only experienced GP present, although individual trainers are often used as a resource.

The content of the course will depend on need as defined by participant trainees and their trainers but will be expected to include subjects less well covered by the undergraduate curriculum or other postgraduate experi-ence, predominantly human behaviour, psychology and interpersonal skills, relationships with other professional and community organizations, the function of primary health care in society, practice organization and the legal and statutory aspects of practice.

Some examples of group activities

Topics – Individual preparation and presentation to group.
Clinical   e.g. Asthma, diabetes, handicapped children, strokes, fits and faints.
Organizational   e.g. Prescribing patterns, home visits, out-of-hours work, GP hospitals.

Journal club and book reviews
e.g.   Individual responsibility for reading a journal, viz. *Update, JRCGP,*

BMJ, informing group and leading a discussion.
Reviewing book and presenting opinion to group.

Case material/prescribing/audit
e.g.   Random case analysis
Problem case analysis
Investigation and referral analysis
Prescription analysis
Creating protocols
Analysing data.

Audiovisual techniques
Consultation analysis – stimulated recall
   – real consultations, simulated consultations, role play and discussion.
Communication skills
Professional material available from: MSD Foundation, BMTV, GPTV, universities, Graves Audio-visual Library, pharmaceutical companies.

Examination techniques
e.g.   MEQs, MCQs, quizzes.

Outside resources
Didactic or semi-didactic teaching and discussion
e.g.   GPs, Clinical Consultants, Community Physicians, Health Visitors, Nurses, Social Workers, pharmacists, Marriage Guidance Counsellors, FPC administrators, CHC, coroners, solicitors, accountants, teachers, architects, research workers, BEA, BDA, police, BMA, MDU.

Sensitivity groups
e.g.   Balint-style, T-Group

Visits
e.g.   Selected practices, Rehabilitation Units, Abortion Clinic, Hospice. FPC, LMC, DRO, DHSS, RCGP, Industrial Medical Centre, Alcoholic Unit, Part III Accommodation, Schools for Handicapped, EBS, GP Relief Service, Day Hospitals, Probation, Social Service Office, pharmaceutical company.

The Trainee Year

Traditionally, trainees spent the whole year with one trainer in one practice. Increasingly, however, trainees in 3-year schemes start with a short initial period of 2–3 months in one practice and complete the last 9–10 months, often in a different practice, 2 years later. Various other combinations have been experimented with and increasingly teaching practices contain more than one appointed trainer.

Nevertheless, certain principles apply whatever the individual arrangements and suggestions are listed below:

1. **Initial assessment of previous experience and present competence by Trainee and Trainer together**
   – curriculum vitae, interview, discussion

- Confidence Rating Scale ⎫
- Manchester Rating Scale ⎬ paper-based or
- MCQs ⎪ microcomputer
- MEQs ⎭

2. **Introduction to practice**
   - ancillary staff, structure, records, forms and certificates
   - attached staff, spend some time with Health Visitors, District Nurses, Midwives, Community Psychiatric Nurses, Social Workers
   - local pharmacist
   - local hospital and Postgraduate Medical Centre

3. **Introduction to consultations and visits**
   - joint consultations and visits with trainer initially
   - conducting surgeries with trainer adjoining, initially with no time constraints
   - out-of-hours work covered by trainer or partners
   - discussion of experience with trainer regularly
   - tutorial sessions

4. **Advice and guidance, re outside resources**
   - trainer/trainee group
   - half-day release course
   - attendance at outpatients, e.g. skins, ENT, eyes
   - Postgraduate Diplomas, e.g. family planning certificate
   - books and journals
   - visits to other practices
   - applying for posts

5. **Project within practice**
   - disease group, hospital referrals, prescribing

6. **Continuing review of progress**
   - adequate clinical experience and discussion time
   - adequate release and study time
   - occasional joint consultation sessions
   - feedback from colleagues, staff and patients

7. **Final evaluation and guidance**
   - Confidence Rating Scale
   - Manchester Rating Scale or similar
   - advise re MRCGP exam
   - advise re career
   - provision of references
   - provision of Certificate of Satisfactory Completion of Training (VTR.I)

Structure of Postgraduate Education for General Practice

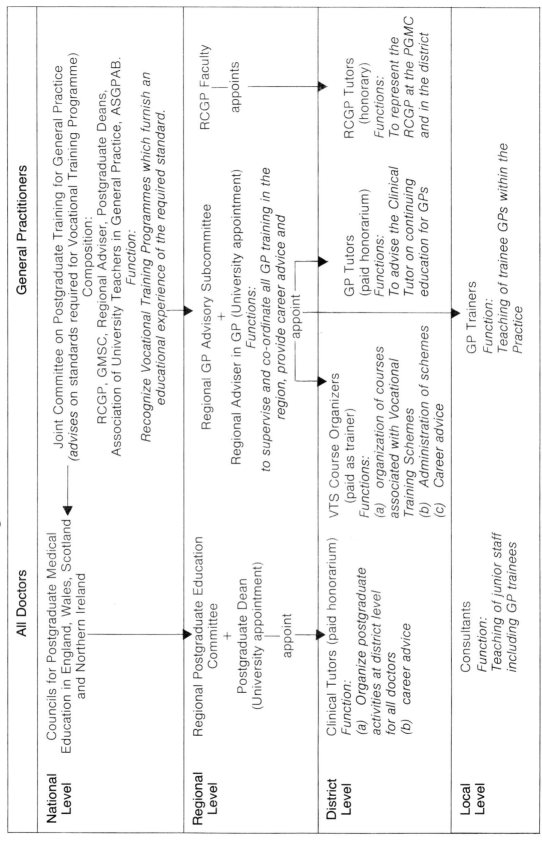

	All Doctors	**General Practitioners**
National Level	Councils for Postgraduate Medical Education in England, Wales, Scotland and Northern Ireland	Joint Committee on Postgraduate Training for General Practice (advises on standards required for Vocational Training Programme) Composition: RCGP, GMSC, Regional Adviser, Postgraduate Deans, Association of University Teachers in General Practice, ASGPAB. Function: Recognize Vocational Training Programmes which furnish an educational experience of the required standard.
Regional Level	Regional Postgraduate Education Committee + Postgraduate Dean (University appointment) appoint	Regional GP Advisory Subcommittee + Regional Adviser in GP (University appointment) Functions: to supervise and co-ordinate all GP training in the region, provide career advice and appoint
District Level	Clinical Tutors (paid honorarium) Function: (a) Organize postgraduate activities at district level for all doctors (b) career advice	VTS Course Organizers (paid as trainer) Functions: (a) organization of courses associated with Vocational Training Schemes (b) Administration of schemes (c) Career advice GP Tutors (paid honorarium) Functions: To advise the Clinical Tutor on continuing education for GPs RCGP Tutors (honorary) Functions: To represent the RCGP at the PGMC and in the district — RCGP Faculty appoints
Local Level	Consultants Function: Teaching of junior staff including GP trainees	GP Trainers Function: Teaching of trainee GPs within the Practice

Criteria for Membership of the Royal College of General Practitioners

Candidates for membership must:

1. be fully registered medical practitioners who have completed, or who will complete within 8 weeks of the date of the oral examination, 3 years' full-time, or equivalent part-time, postregistration experience which:

    (a) includes not less than 2 years in general practice (including any periods as a trainee practitioner),

    or

    (b) consists of a special postregistration programme of vocational training for general practice recognized by the College

    or

    (c) ensures eligibility for the JCPTGP's Certificate of prescribed or equivalent experience.

2. pass the examination in accordance with Ordinance 3 of the Royal Charter.

The MRCGP Examination

The College examination is at present in two parts.

Part 1 consists of:
A Modified Essay Question paper (MEQ) (1 hour)
A Practice Topic Question paper (PTQ) (2 hours)
A Multiple Choice Question paper (MCQ) (2 hours).

Part 2 consists of two consecutive oral examinations held approximately 6 weeks after Part 1.

This examination is based on the job description of the general practitioner and the educational aims of vocational training as set out by a working party appointed by the Second European Conference on the Teaching of General Practice (*see* pp. 113–114). The knowledge, skills and attitudes exhibited by the candidate are assessed in a variety of ways in different parts of the examination, as follows.

Clinical practice – health and disease. The candidate will be required to demonstrate a knowledge of the diagnosis, management and, where appropriate, the prevention of diseases of importance in general practice:

    (a) The range of the normal
    (b) The patterns of illness
    (c) The natural history of diseases
    (d) Prevention
    (e) Early diagnosis
    (f) Diagnostic methods and techniques
    (g) Management and treatment

Clinical practice – human development. The candidate will be expected to possess a knowledge of human development and be able to demonstrate the value of this knowledge in the diagnosis and management of patients in general practice.

(a)   Genetics
(b)   Fetal development
(c)   Physical development in childhood, maturity and ageing
(d)   Intellectual development in childhood, maturity and ageing
(e)   Emotional development in childhood, maturity and ageing
(f)   The range of the normal

Clinical practice – human behaviour. The candidate must demonstrate an understanding of human behaviour particularly as it affects the presentation and management of disease.

(a)   Behaviour presenting to the general practitioner
(b)   Behaviour in interpersonal relationships
(c)   Behaviour of the family
(d)   Behaviour in the doctor–patient relationship

Medicine and society. The candidate must be familiar with the common sociological and epidemiological concepts and their relevance to medical care, and demonstrate a knowledge of the organization of medical and related services in the United Kingdom and abroad.

(a)   Sociological aspects of health and ilness
(b)   The uses of epidemiology
(c)   The organization of medical care in the UK – comparisons with other countries.
(d)   The relationship of medical services to other institutions of society

The practice. The candidate must demonstrate a knowledge of practice organization and administration and be able to critically discuss recent developments in the evolution of general practice.

(a)   Practice management
(b)   The Team
(c)   Financial matters
(d)   Premises and equipment
(e)   Medical records
(f)   Medicolegal matters
(g)   Research

The examination is designed to assess in a variety of ways the skills of the candidate:

In interpersonal communication
In history taking and information gathering
In selecting examinations using investigations and procedures
In recording information
In interpreting information
In problem definition and hypothesis formation
In early diagnosis
In defining the range of intervention
In selecting therapy
In providing continuing care
In interventive and preventive medicine in relation to:
    (a)   the patient
    (b)   the family
    (c)   the community
In the organization of his practice and himself
In teamwork, delegation, and in relating to other colleagues

In business methods

In communications

The candidate will be expected to demonstrate appropriate attitudes to his patients, to his colleagues and to the role of the general practitioner. He must demonstrate his ability to develop and extend his knowledge and skills through continuing education.

A candidate may elect to sit Part 1 in one of several centres; currently London, Birmingham, Leeds, Manchester, Newcastle, Edinburgh, Aberdeen, Cardiff, Belfast and Dublin.

The oral examinations are held only in London and Edinburgh.

Further details about the College and the Examination may be obtained from:

The Examination Administrator,
Royal College of General Practitioners,
14 Princes Gate,
Hyde Park,
London SW7 1PU.

Continuing Education

Continuing education for established general practitioners has been generously supported by the DHSS, through Section 63 funding, and by the pharmaceutical companies. Unfortunately, although the volume of educational material offered has been enormous, the quality and content has not been as carefully devised or evaluated as has that provided for vocational training. General practitioners are taking increasing responsibility for their own continuing education and many small groups have been formed, especially by younger practitioners, for mutual support, discussion, educational and research activities.

Listed below are some of the facilities available.

District Postgraduate Centres
Lunchtime, sessional or extended courses
Library facilities
Advice and help from Clinical Tutors, GP Tutors and the Postgraduate Secretary
Learning methods used include: lectures, group work, studies and investigations, audiovisual facilities

Regional and National Centres
Day, extended and intensive courses
For availability refer to:
Postgraduate Secretary
Regional Postgraduate Organization booklets
Journal advertising

Royal College of General Practitioners
Refer to Courses Secretary

Clinical Assistantships
Dependent on local availability

Clinical Attachments
Personal arrangement via Regional Postgraduate Adviser in GP

Prolonged study leave
See Statements of Fees and Allowances (Red Book)

MD thesis
Apply to qualifying university for advice

Funding organizations
For help with research, travel, etc.
  DHSS
  Regional Health Authority
  Nuffield Provincial Hospitals Trust
  King's Fund
  Pharmaceutical companies
  Medical Research Council

Practice activities
Developing management protocols
Audit methods
— prescribing
— deaths
— serious illness
— emergencies
— hospital referrals
Journal club
Multidisciplinary meetings

Section C

EMERGENCIES

Acute Abdomen

What might it be:

Sudden   ○ abdominal pain
             ○ vomiting
             ○ bowel change
             ○ bleeding
             ○ shock/collapse

face the GP with a potential life/death situation.

The rate of acute abdomen in a typical practice of 2500 may be:

acute appendicitis	3 cases every year
renal colic	2 cases every year
biliary colic	1 case every year
intestinal obstruction	1 case every year
peptic ulcer complications	1 case every year
strangulated hernia	1 case every 2 years
acute pancreatitis	1 case every 4 years
ectopic pregnancy	1 case every 4 years
gynae emergencies	1 case every 4 years
diverticulitis	1 case every 5 years
congenital pyloric stenosis, etc.	1 case every 10 years

after Fry. J. 'Common Diseases' (1983)

The **problems** facing the GP are:
○ has the patient an acute surgical abdomen?
○ should immediate hospital admission be arranged?
○ if not: what further investigations should be done?
           should a specialist opinion be arranged?
           when should the patient be seen again?
○   what should the patient/family be told?

Assessment:

History
○ pain   — how long
                         — where
                         — what character
                         — has it moved
○ vomit   — how many times
                         — character
○ bowels   — last open
                         — diarrhoea
                         — appearance
○ micturition   — any change
○ menses   — LMP
                         — discharge
                         — on pill
○ other symptoms   — ?
○ previous history   — similar attack
                         — operations
                         — major illnesses
○ family history   — ?

Examination

○ abdomen — follow sequential pattern
 — (do not forget groins, scrotum, vagina, rectum)
 — look before you feel
 — palpate gently for tenderness, rebound and guarding
○ TPR — take and note
○ urine — infected
 — blood
 — sugar
 — porphyria
○ throat — acute throat infection as cause of abdominal pain in child
○ chest — non-surgical causes of acute abdominal pain, i.e. pneumonia, myocardial infarction, ruptured aorta.

NOTE: abdominal pain lasting more than 3–4 hours is likely to be an acute abdomen

child who can jump up and down is unlikely to have acute abdomen

beware, we have all missed the occasional acute abdomen.

The role of the GP is **not** to make a **definite diagnosis,** which must always be retrospective.

Clinical pointers
○ acute appendicitis is chiefly a condition of young adults but can occur at any age.

○ renal colic is often recurrent, but is more common in men.

○ biliary colic is more common in women, the pain is worse than labour pain and is becoming more prevalent.

○ intestinal obstruction is secondary to some primary mechanical causes which are more likely in the elderly.

○ ectopic pregnancy is becoming more frequent, note women with IUD.

Do not delay, see patient quickly.
Remember the **sins of clinical omission** and follow recognized sequence of
○ history
○ examination
○ assessment
○ discussion with patient/family.

If **acute abdomen is likely,** then:
○ arrange immediate hospital admission

If **acute abdomen is possible,** then:
○ arrange for immediate hospital admission
 or
○ arrange for immediate domiciliary consultation
 or
○ arrange for immediate hospital O.P. assessment
 or
○ arrange to see the patient in a few, 2–3 hours
 DO NOT LEAVE OVERNIGHT

If **acute abdomen is unlikely,** then:
○ arrange to see the patient again soon
○ instruct patient/family to report any change or deterioration.

Anaphylaxis

What might it be:
Immediate systemic reaction to antigen (reagin) entering sensitized person by –
- injection –   penicillin, foreign sera or insect bites
therapeutic desensitization, etc.
- ingestion –   drugs, e.g. penicillin or aspirin
foods, e.g. shellfish
- inhalation –   pollens, animal dander

Effects

General
- collapse, convulsions, coma
- fall in BP
- tachycardia – cardiac arrest – death
- shock
- anuria
- coma

Respiratory
- laryngeal oedema
- bronchospasm
- pulmonary oedema

GI tract
- vomiting
- diarrhoea

Skin
- angioneurotic oedema
- urticaria
- maculopapular rash
- pruritus

Assessment:
- one of the most urgent and life threatening situations in practice
- may be immediate result of obvious injection or may be delayed after ingestion of food or drug
- history – what has been injected or taken
    - previous history
    - Medic-Alert disc/bracelet

What is it:
- diagnosis of anaphylaxis is usually obvious
- no time to waste in endeavouring to pinpoint causal factors – the management is the same for all.

What to do:
- lay in head down–feet up position
- clear air passages
- insert airway if necessary
- inject adrenaline (1:1000) slowly 0.5 ml s.c.
repeat every 5 minutes if necessary
- inject hydrocortisone hemisuccinate 100 mg i.v.
- CPR if required

Back Pain

What might it be:

More than 9 out of 10 acute backs have no serious underlying cause and recover with simple measures within 2–3 weeks.
Acute backs tend to recur. They are most frequent in 30–60 age group.

Possible more serious causes
O prolapsed intervertebral disc
O vertebral collapse secondary to
     – neoplasia (usually secondaries)
     – osteoporosis
     – trauma
     – infection (TB)

Assessment:

History
O causal incident – often minor
O previous history – recurrences common
O radiation ⟶ leg (sciatica)
O aggravating factors – cough, strain
O bladder function
O sensory symptoms

Examination
O back   – movements
                 – tenderness
O sacro-iliacs
O straight leg raise
O reflexes   – knee
                 – ankle
                 – plantar
O sensation   – leg
                 – perineum
O motor   – power
                 – wasting
O abdomen
O rectal }
O pelvic } if indicated

Investigations
Unnecessary in majority of attacks
If no improvement after 2–3 weeks (or other indications)
O X-Rays of back and chest
O FBC and ESR
     O if Ca prostate suspected – serum acid phosphatase
     O if myelomatosis suspected
          O electrophoresis
          O Bence Jones proteinuria

What is it:

Assume it is a **'minor non-specific acute back'** unless –
O radiation down leg and SLR limited
O severe pain with local tenderness
O bladder function disturbed
O persists and recurs + +
O definite evidence of neurological damage,
   e.g. diminished reflexes, anaesthetic areas

What to do: Most begin to settle in 2–3 days with:
○ strict bed rest on boards
○ analgesics
    ○ aspirin/paracetamol usually adequate ± muscle relaxant, e.g. diazepam
If no improvement
○ re-assess and investigate
○ consider epidural injection
○ consider manipulation
○ consider corset support

If severe and prolonged then –
○ refer to consultant
    ○ domiciliary consultation
    ○ OPD
○ assess personal–family problems
○ admit urgently to hospital if any signs or symptoms of central disc prolapse found, e.g.
    bilateral nerve root pressure
    disturbance of micturition
    perineal anaesthesia
THIS IS A SURGICAL EMERGENCY

Bereavement

**What might
it be:**

Grief is a normal reaction to bereavement but can sometimes be severe and overwhelming and the sufferer may need care and protection at various times.

Various stages of grieving are described but they may not all occur nor necessarily in the order shown and may overlap.

- Shock with disbelief, denial, numbness or blunting. The person may appear to be unaffected by the death
- Fear-like symptoms/panic attacks
- Distress with weeping and feelings of physical pain
- Searching, associated with disbelief
- 'Finding' or a feeling of nearness. There may be hallucinations or illusions of the dead person being present
- Anger and guilt – both self and others may be blamed. Trivial events in the past assume great importance
- Physical symptoms – sometimes mimic the dead person's symptoms: sometimes associated with anxiety
- Depression
- Feelings of inadequacy
- Readjustment – finding a new identity

Assessment:

The severity and length of these symptoms is extremely variable and it is difficult to decide when a normal grief reaction has become a pathological one.

Excessively severe or prolonged symptoms from which there is apparently no progress may constitute an abnormal reaction and need special help.

What to do:

○ Bereaved people need help and support. If family, friends or neighbours are present, there may be little need for anyone else.
○ Help and support may be sought and should always be offered, by the practice team at the beginning and at intervals throughout the first 2 years following. Planned provision of care may prevent morbidity.
○ Encourage them to talk as much as necessary and to cry whenever they need to.
○ Confirm that the awful feelings they are experiencing are normal in the circumstances, and will persist for a long time.
○ Praise the care they gave the deceased.
○ Arrange a follow up appointment.

What *not* to do:

○ Never say 'you will get over it eventually'. This implies that they will forget the dead person and they do not want to do that.
○ Never prescribe tranquillizers or hypnotics. If you feel unable to refuse, limit provision to one or two from a stock of your own.

Bleeding

**What might
it be:**

Observed: the patient presents as bleeding.
Concealed: the patient presents as shocked, breathless, having fainted and with pain or discomfort at the site of the bleeding.

Assessment:

Assessment of the amount of blood loss by the history is unreliable: vaginal bleeding always seems more than it is and gastrointestinal bleeding less. BUT it is not safe to wait until there are symptoms or signs of shock before admitting a bleeding patient to hospital. *Bleeding is frightening* and a doctor may be called for bleeding which is in fact insignificant, e.g.

○ Slight haemoptysis in association with a URTI is usually due to blood coming from the postnasal space
○ A streak of blood in the vomit of a posseting infant with a URTI usually originates from the postnasal space
○ Streaks of blood on the motions of a bottle fed baby are common and unimportant

Site
Observed:

○ **Nose** – epistaxes are unimportant in children and young adults unless especially heavy and prolonged. In the elderly, more care is needed
○ **Upper gastrointestinal tract** – haematemesis and melaena are always important (unless the merest streak)
   Has it happened before recently?
   Is it accompanied by melaena?
○ **Rectal** – fresh or altered
   Melaena always serious and urgent
   Fresh blood may be serious but not necessarily need emergency investigation
○ **Haemoptysis**
   Important if repeated or more than a streak in association with a URTI
   Rarely needs emergency treatment
○ **Vaginal**
   Important in pregnancy or puerperium or post abortion (its absence does not exclude an ectopic pregnancy)
   Excessive menstrual loss may need emergency treatment

Concealed:
Common in haemophiliacs.
Intracranial:
   extradural
   subdural
   subarachnoid
   cerebral

Thoracic
Abdominal: always significant

What is it:

Haematemesis and melaena
Oesophageal varices
Peptic ulcer
Acute gastric erosion
Carcinoma

History of repeated recent haematemasis with or without melaena may mean that the patient is already depleted and anaemic. Melaena may be diagnosed by the characteristic smell on entering the house even in the absence of a clearcut history. (Beware of oral iron producing black stools imitating melaena but without the characteristic smell.)

Rectal bleeding (other than melaena)
Carcinoma
Diverticular disease
Ulcerative colitis
Proctitis
Piles

Haemoptysis
Always needs to be investigated but usually no urgency and often no cause found.
○ Common in chronic bronchitis
○ Cancer
○ TB
○ Aortic aneurysm eroding into bronchus – rare and usually rapidly fatal

Vaginal
○ In pregnancy
    Before 28 weeks – threatened abortion.
        Ectopic pregnancy may cause symptoms before a missed period or before pregnancy has been confirmed. Classically pain precedes vaginal bleeding but this is not reliable. There may be no vaginal loss.
    After 28 weeks – APH – revealed accidental haemorrhage
                            placenta praevia
                            premature labour
○ After pregnancy, ERPC or STOP, secondary haemorrhage may be due to retained products or to infection.
○ Menstrual bleeding may be excessive due to metropathia, IUCD, carcinoma, uterine polyp or to no identifiable cause.
○ Intermenstrual bleeding may be due to forgotten OC pill, carcinoma of cervix, cervical erosion, cervical polyps.

Concealed (internal) bleeding
In haemophiliacs, acute pain and swelling in muscles or joints is a common presentation of haemorrhage.

Intracranial:
    extradural – soon after head injury
    subdural – delayed after head injury
    subarachnoid – spontaneous from berry aneurysm
    cerebral – stroke

Intrathoracic (rare): ruptured ventricular or aortic aneurysm, usually immediately fatal.

Intra-abdominal
○ Ruptured spleen, liver, kidney – usually history of injury in UK
○ Aortic aneurysm – bleeding may start slowly and be retroperitoneal causing backache

What to do:

Admit at once:
Haematemesis and melaena

Threatened abortion with heavy bleeding
APH
Suspected ectopic pregnancy
Intra-abdominal bleeding
Extradural, subdural and subarachnoid haemorrhages

Consider admission:
Elderly with persistent epistaxis
Secondary haemorrhage after pregnancy

Acute severe blood loss
○ Lie in head-down position
○ Set up i.v. fluids (if available) – take blood for cross-matching first
○ Morphine 15 mg s.c.
○ Control bleeding site if possible
○ Flying squad summoned (if available)
○ Urgent admission (hospital alerted)

Blindness

○ usually unilateral

What might it be:

Distinguish
○ sudden onset of blindness
○ sudden discovery of blindness by patient

Possible causes
○ glaucoma (acutely painful)
○ cataract (progressive)
○ migraine (transient)
○ senile macular degeneration (gradual)
○ retinal detachment (sudden)
○ giant cell arteritis (sudden)
○ multiple sclerosis
○ intracranial neoplasm
○ central retinal artery occlusion (sudden)
○ malignant hypertension
○ central retinal vein occlusion (sudden)
○ macular haemorrhages (sudden)
○ carotid artery occlusion
○ methanol drinking
○ hysteria

Assessment:

Check
○ visual acuity
○ visual fields
○ systematic examination of eyes
○ other systems
    ○ CVS
    ○ CNS
    ○ urine
    ○ ESR

What to do:

Arrange for urgent consultation with consultant ophthalmologist.

Breathlessness

What might it be:

Common
○ Left ventricular failure
○ Asthma
○ Acute on chronic obstructive airways disease (COAD)

Less common:
○ Spontaneous pneumothorax (may complicate asthma or COAD)
○ Pulmonary embolism
○ Hysterical hyperventilation
○ Pneumonia
○ Inhaled foreign body
○ Laryngeal obstruction – foreign body; oedema

Assessment:

Left ventricular failure is more likely in older patient and asthma in the very young, but asthma may occur for first time in middle age.

History may reveal previous similar attacks, their treatment and outcome (but beware pneumothorax in a known asthmatic).

Ask about recent
  - orthopnoea
  - shortness of breath on exertion
  - chest pain and type – cardiac, pleuritic?
  - drug treatment (β-blockers may precipitate asthma or left ventricular failure)
  - sputum character

Examination: observe position and general condition while taking history
  - central cyanosis
  - difficulty speaking
  - prolonged expiration
  - peripheral circulation
  - pulse – rate, character
  - JVP
  - sacral/ankle oedema
  - liver
  - blood pressure
  - chest movements and percussion note
  - auscultation – often unhelpful: the chest sounds wheezy in both left ventricular failure and asthma. In severe asthma the chest is silent. Reduced apical air entry may be the only sign of a pneumothorax

What is it:

	Asthma/COAD	Left ventricular failure
History	Previous attacks	Previous attacks
	Nocturnal cough	Hypertension
	Recent URTI	Ischaemic heart disease
	Allergic contact	Valvular disease
	Emotional crisis	β-blockers
	Purulent sputum	Anginal pain
		Orthopnoea
		Frothy sputum ± blood flecks
Examination	Reduced respiratory movement	Tachycardia with weak pulse
	Hyperinflated chest	Widespread fine creps. and wheezing or **no** chest signs or basal creps only
	Prolonged expiration ± wheeze	
	Central cyanosis	
	Tachycardia	Signs of RHF (JVP▲) oedema Liver +

Asthma:

Severe	**Less severe**
Unable to talk	Talks
Unable to use peak flow meter	Peak flow 150 or more
Quiet chest	Good colour
Tachycardia over 120	Loud expiratory wheeze
Restlessness or confusion	Pulse rate less than 110

What to do:

Asthma:
Severe
○ Hydrocortisone i.v. 200 mg stat (**or** prednisolone 40 mg orally)
○ Admit to hospital immediately requesting oxygen in ambulance and no delay.
○ Salbutamol 250 μg i.v. slowly } or twice dose
  or terbutaline 250 μg i.v. slowly } s.c.
  or aminophylline 250 mg (10 ml) very slowly
       (**not** if patient has been taking oral aminophylline or theophylline)
○ In children, use half all above-listed doses

Less severe
○ Salbutamol 5 mg in 5 ml ± ipratropium 500 μg (40 drops) in nebulizer (half doses in children)

○ Prednisolone 20 mg stat by mouth (and then q.d.s. in reducing doses)
Provide peak flow meter to monitor progress.
If no improvement after 1 hour, admit to hospital.
If improves, beware relapse when effect of nebulizer wears off.
If possible, leave nebulizer with patient to be used every 3–4 hours.

Mild
No previous treatment: salbutamol by inhaler.
Already on treatment: check inhalers correctly used: review total medication; add inhaled steroid if necessary.

Left ventricular failure:
○ Sit up with legs down.
○ Diamorphine 5 mg i.v. + 5 mg i.m. (as long as sure of diagnosis)
○ Frusemide 40 mg i.v. followed by oral dose
○ Aminophylline 250 mg i.v. (very slowly and only if no oral aminophylline or theophylline taken)
○ Oxygen if available.
○ Review medication (stop β-blocker)

Response is usually dramatic unless complicating infarct or arrhythmia.
Admit to hospital if cannot be managed at home or other complicating factor.
If in doubt about diagnosis give frusemide and aminophylline.

Chest Pain

What might it be: Only central (retrosternal) chest pain is likely to present as an emergency:
- Myocardial infarction
- Pericarditis
- Angina
- Dissecting aortic aneurysm
- Pulmonary embolism
- Indigestion – reflux oesophagitis, gastritis
- Costochondritis
- Referred pain from cervical or thoracic spine

Assessment:

History
Family history (e.g. of ischaemic heart disease at early age)
Age
Lifestyle including personality, smoking habits, build, exercise
Description of the pain:
- is this the first time?
- onset
- character
- site and radiation
- duration
- severity
- accompanying symptoms
- effect of position, exercise
- relieving factors
- exacerbating or precipitating factors
- medication

What does the patient think it is?

Examination
General condition – probably frightened
Colour
Pulse – rate, character
Blood pressure
JVP, liver, oedema
Heart – size, character of impulse
Chest, including costochondral junctions
Spine, especially neck

Investigations
Electrocardiogram may not be able to confirm the diagnosis **but** if taken while the pain is present and if normal, the pain is most unlikely to be ischaemic.

What is it:

Myocardial infarction
- Pain central/retrosternal, severe, crushing or constricting
- May radiate to neck, jaw, arms
- Usually lasts half an hour or more
- May be associated with dyspnoea, shock, nausea

(But beware the 'silent infarct' in the elderly)

Pulmonary embolism
- May be indistinguishable from myocardial infarction
- Dyspnoea

○ Cough
○ Haemoptysis
○ Pleuritic pain
○ Source of embolus, e.g. postoperative, postpartum, deep vein thrombosis

Dissecting aneurysm
○ May be indistinguishable from myocardial infarction
○ Sudden onset, severe pain, often through to back
○ Peripheral pulses may be absent

What to do: Diamorphine 5 mg i.v. stat mixed with cyclizine 50 mg instead of water. A further 5 mg diamorphine i.m. may be needed to produce continued relief or cover journey to hospital.

Myocardial infarction
Admit to hospital if patient
○ has arrhythmia
○ is young
○ would prefer it
○ lives alone

Consider home care if
○ patient in good condition
○ long interval since episode of pain
○ patient over 65 years
○ domestic and nursing arrangements allow it
○ patient and family happy about it

Consider hospital admission after a delay if the patient is shocked

Home care
○ Bed rest until free from pain, then limited mobility (no stairs) for 10 days
○ Light meals
○ No smoking
○ E.c.g.
○ Cardiac enzymes } within 48 hours
○ Watch for arrhythmias, heart failure
○ Mobilize gradually
○ Advise on return to work, lifestyle, smoking, diet

Croup

What might it be:
○ Acute laryngitis with stridor
○ Majority are associated with viral or *H.influenzae* upper respiratory tract infections
○ Affects children between 6 months and 4 years
○ Other rare causes are epiglottitis, diphtheria, inhaled foreign body, trauma, papilloma and angioneurotic oedema

Assessment:
○ Usually at night
○ Parents and child frightened
○ Best assessed after a few minutes quiet chat when the panic has subsided
○ Mild attack:
   – the stridor goes when the child (and parents) calm down, and is replaced by an intermittent rasping cough
   – child remains alert, good colour and muscle tone
○ Severe attack:
   – stridor continues with each inspiration
   – child limp, ashen or cyanosed

What is it:
○ Assume upper respiratory tract infection cause unless otherwise indicated

What to do:
Admit to hospital if:
○ Severe attack which persists
○ Parents unable to cope either through panic or inadequacy

Home care:
○ Reassurance and explanation
○ Warm drinks and warm, steamy atmosphere
○ Amoxycillin if child under 1 year

Death – Sudden and Unexpected

What might it be:

In any year in the UK

Total deaths	600 000
Deaths in hospital	350 000
Deaths outside hospital	250 000
Sudden and unexpected deaths (Reported to Coroner)	60 000 (2 per GP)

Sudden and unexpected deaths – causes   %

	%
Ischaemic coronary heart disease	55
Other heart disease	9
Pulmonary embolism	6
Ruptured aortic aneurysm	6
Acute respiratory disease	7
Cot deaths	2
Acute abdomen	2
Suicide	5
Road traffic accident	5
Others	3
(After H. G. Penman, in Scientific Foundations of Family Medicine, 1978)	100

Assessment:

- confirm death
- establish identity
- history from witnesses
- examine body

What is it:

- almost all sudden deaths are from natural causes
- once in a professional lifetime you will meet an un-natural cause – be prepared!

What to do:

- if deceased had medical care in past 14 days – possible for doctor who saw patient alive to issue death certificate if satisfied of cause of death
- if no medical attention in past 14 days – notify the coroner's officer (via police)
- notify the coroner's officer if –
    - accident, injury or operation in past year
    - uncertain causes
    - allegations of negligence
    - alcoholism/self-neglect
    - war or industrial disability pension
    - result of medical/surgical treatment
    - suicide
    - in prison/custody

(In Scotland Procurator-Fiscal acts as Coroner)
- support family – explain and inform
- removal of body (by local undertakers)
- if autopsy – try to attend

Dental and Oral

What might it be:

Pain
- toothache, ulceration, abscess

Bleeding
- post-extraction haemorrhage

Ulceration
- aphthous, herpetic, Vincent's angina

Swelling
- trauma, infection, salivary glands, allergy

Assessment:

History
- dental, medication, systemic illness

Examination
- general
- local
  - mucous membranes, tongue, gums
    teeth, extraction sites
    salivary glands

Diagnosis and management:

Dental caries or pulpitis
- analgesics, refer dentist

Dental abscess
- antibiotics, analgesics, refer dentist

Dental haemorrhage (post-extraction)
- remove clot
- bite on folded gauze or handkerchief
- if not controlled will need suture

Aphthous ulceration
- analgesics, mouthwashes

Vincent's angina
- penicillin, metronidazole

Diarrhoea and Vomiting

What might it be:

Acute D & V is endemic and affects all ages.
Acute D & V is potentially dangerous in infants because of secondary interference with water and electrolyte balance.

Causes of acute D & V are uncertain. In only a small minority definable pathogenic bacteria (*E. coli,* dysentery, typhoid–paratyphoid, cholera and food poisoning organism, protozoa (giardiasis) or viruses (rota viruses) detectable.
It must be assumed that at present most D & V in practice is of uncertain cause.

NOTE: D & V may occur in association with remote infections (in children) such as acute otitis media.
– as part of acute abdomen – appendicitis, intussuseption, and mesenteric artery thrombosis.
– with malabsorption syndrome.

Assessment:

History
O possible food poisoning
O other cases in family (or area)
O recent travel overseas
O duration
O severity – vomit/diarrhoea
O other symptoms in other systems
O ? food handler

Examination
O general condition
O TPR
O dehydration (look at tongue, fontanelle, tissue turgor)
O abdominal examination:
        O tenderness
        O distension
        O masses
O rectal examination if indicated
O ears
O throat } in children
O chest
O inspect vomit
O inspect faeces

Investigations are normally unhelpful but essential in food handlers, possible food poisoning, severe cases or following overseas travel.

Faeces should be examined for organisms etc. if condition lasts more than a few days and if epidemic present.

What to do:

Majority of D & V settle naturally within 2–3 days.
There is no need for antibiotics or any other medication.

General advice
O no solids to be eaten
O plentiful fluids by mouth
O small amounts and frequently if vomiting

○ since attacks tend to be over in 2–3 days no need for special formulation of fluid

Infants
○ NO solids
○ continue breast-feeding
○ ½ strength milk in mild attacks
○ glucose–electrolyte mixture 1–2 hourly in infants under 6 months

NOTE: lactose intolerance in recurrent or persistent diarrhoea

If no improvement in 2–3 days:

Children and adults: reconsider diagnosis – faecal examination
Infants: consider hospital admission to correct dehydration

Earache

What might it be:

Children
- ○ acute otitis media (the most usual cause)
- ○ foreign body
- ○ external otitis (rare in children)

Adults
- ○ acute otitis media
- ○ acute/chronic otitis media
- ○ external otitis
- ○ dry hard wax
- ○ referred pain from –
  - ○ dental causes
  - ○ throat infection
  - ○ neuralgia

Assessment:

Ears
- ○ external ear
  - ○ swelling of walls
  - ○ boil
  - ○ dermatitis
  - ○ foreign body
  - ○ wax
- ○ ear drum
  (if there is external otitis or wax it may not be possible to visualize drum and it may be too painful to remove wax)
  - ○ normal
  - ○ red

Mouth
- ○ dental state
- ○ tonsils
- ○ buccal ulcers

General
- ○ degree of illness
  - ○ TPR
  - ○ severity of pain

What is it:

NOTE: infants and young children do not complain of 'earache'.
Present as sick feverish child with abdominal pains.

- ○ examination of ears will reveal –
  - ○ cause in ears
  - ○ no cause in ears
  - ○ consider referred pain

What to do:

Acute otitis media
- ○ more than one half have non-bacterial causes (? viral)
- ○ most likely bacterial causes
  - ○ pneumococci
  - ○ *H. influenzae*
  - ○ *Strep. pyogenes*
- ○ much less dangerous condition than in past
  - ○ less virulent organisms

○ more healthy children
○ many attacks will resolve completely without antibiotics
○ relieve pain with adequate analgesics (e.g. soluble aspirin, paracetamol)
○ reassess in 1–2 days
  ○ if earache improved continue to observe and follow-up. (Ear drum will take up to 3 weeks to return to normal.)
  ○ if earache still present and child unwell give –
    ○ penicillin V
  or ○ amoxycillin
  or ○ ampicillin
  or ○ co-trimoxazole
  ○ essential to follow-up until drum and hearing return to normal

Acute otitis externa

○ if localized boil (furuncle)
  ○ oral antibiotics
○ if diffuse dermatitis
  ○ cleanse out meatus
  ○ steroid-antibiotic eardrops
○ antibiotics by mouth } in severe cases
○ steroids by mouth

Falls

What might it be:

○ Most will go straight to Accident and Emergency Department
○ Likely to be seen by GP at home:
    – elderly
    – drunks
    – children

○ Watch for
    – fractured neck of femur
    – head injuries
    – ruptured spleen
    – non-accidental injury (*see* p.156)

Assessment:

Fractured neck of femur

○ Most common in elderly women
○ Fall may have been minor
○ Symptoms may be minimal
○ Usually unable to walk but some can walk immediately after if the fracture is impacted
○ Lies with leg in external rotation
○ Rotational movements of leg limited and painful

Head injuries, neck injuries, ruptured spleen

○ Common in drunks who fall downstairs at home
○ May be unconscious or confused because of drink
○ Symptoms and signs unreliable
○ Beware those who cannot be roused and made to co-operate and walk
○ Watch for extradural haemorrhage during first 24 hours, subdural during the following weeks

What to do:

○ May not be possible to sort out at home
○ If in doubt send to Accident and Emergency Department or observe for a few hours

Fits, Faints, Convulsions

What might it be:

In a **child** or **young adult:**
○ vasovagal attack
○ epileptic fit or febrile convulsion
○ hysteria

In an **elderly person:**
○ vasovagal attack
○ epileptic fit
○ transient ischaemic attack
○ Stokes–Adams attack

In an **insulin-dependent diabetic:**
○ hypoglycaemia

Assessment:

History: most important as the attack has usually finished by the time the doctor arrives.
– age
– previous similar attack
– medication; alcohol
– description of attack by patient and by eyewitness

Examination:
– level of consciousness, general behaviour, affect, memory
– evidence of incontinence, injury, tongue biting
– focal neurological signs
– pulse – quality, rate
– blood pressure
– in a child:
   ○ fever and causes for it, e.g. otitis media, tonsillitis, prodromal measles (look for Koplik's spots)
   ○ meningism: neck stiffness, Kernig's

What is it:

Vasovagal attack	Epileptic fit
Patient feels faint before	No warning but specific aura occasionally
Nausea common	
No aura	No nausea
Pallor	Good colour
Slow, weak pulse	Strong pulse
Limp	Convulsive movements and/or grimaces
No movements	
No incontinence	Incontinence common
Alert after	Sleepy after

Transient ischaemic attack likely to be preceded or followed by transient neurological symptoms or signs such as dysarthria, visual disturbance, ataxia, weakness in face or limb.

Stokes–Adams attack: pulse absent or very slow at time of attack and a while after but may be normal by the time the doctor arrives.

Febrile convulsion in child
○ A young infant with meningitis may have no neck stiffness or other physical signs of meningism.
○ Feverish children may be twitchy before having a fit.

What to do:	**Vasovagal attacks:** reassure, advise.

Febrile convulsion in child:

– Admit to hospital if
○ in doubt about cause of fever
○ any suspicion of meningism
○ parents panic-stricken or inadequate

– Treat at home
○ cause of fever obvious
○ convulsion and twitching absent when seen
○ parents calm and sensible

– If still fitting
○ lie on side
○ free airway
○ use wooden spatula or spoon between teeth
○ diazepam (0.5% solution: 5 mg/ml) i.v. slowly, 200 μg/kg i.e. 2 mg for 10 kg child (12–18 months)
  or
  rectally 5 mg age 1–3; 10 mg over 3 years

– Reduce fever
○ fluids
○ tepid sponging
○ aspirin
○ advise parents to avoid excessive clothing and room temperature

– Treat infection if necessary

○ **Transient ischaemic attacks**
  – explain and reassure
  – consider aspirin 75 mg daily
  – arrange follow-up and further investigation if necessary

○ **Stokes–Adams attack**
  – admit if pulse still slow
  – explain and reassure
  – arrange further investigations and possible pacing

Headaches

What might it be:

Common:
○ psychogenic (tension)
○ migrainous
○ toxic

Rare
○ meningitis
○ raised intracranial pressure
○ post-traumatic
○ local pathology — skull, spine, orbits, sinuses, etc
○ subarachnoid
○ temporal arteritis
○ neuralgia

Assessment:

History
○ age
○ family history
○ past medical history — known migraine, hypertension, previous head injury, etc
○ medication
○ depressed/anxious
○ recent symptoms, e.g. fever, malaise, nausea
○ change in personality
○ site of headache
○ onset
○ duration
○ accompanying symptoms — visual disturbances, etc.

Examination
○ general behaviour
○ level of consciousness
○ signs of injury
○ blood pressure, pulse
○ temperature
○ respiratory rate
○ scalp
○ neck ridigity
○ eyes — pupils, fundi
○ signs of focal neurological lesion
○ temporal arteries
○ sinuses

What is it:

Psychogenic
○ described as severe, continuous sense of pressure or tightness
○ usually over vault, less frequently occipito-frontal
○ worse under stress
○ look for symptoms of depression
    ○ loss of weight
    ○ sleep disturbance
    ○ libido, etc.

Migraine
○ recurrent episodes lasting 2 hours to 2 days

- ○ usually unilateral
- ○ photophobia, nausea, vomiting
- ○ aura – usually visual disturbances
- ○ paraesthesiae at angle of mouth or hand
- ○ precipitated by certain foods, contraceptive pill, alcohol, etc.

Meningitis
- ○ pyrexia
- ○ photophobia
- ○ nausea vomiting
- ○ neck rigidity

Raised intracranial pressure
- ○ raised blood pressure
- ○ tumour – slow pulse
- ○ abscess – vomiting
- ○ haematoma – signs of focal lesion common on waking worsened by coughing, sneezing, straining, throbbing, bursting in character
- ○ sometimes worse on lying down
- ○ papilloedema
- ○ visual impairment is late feature

Post-traumatic
- ○ severe, continuous, poorly localized
- ○ made worse by exertion, noise, emotion
- ○ giddiness
- ○ inability to concentrate
- ○ most likely to occur if original injury trivialized
- ○ following lumbar puncture

Extracranial causes
- ○ acute and chronic sinusitis
- ○ eye disease – glaucoma, iridocyclitis
- ○ cervical spondylosis
- ○ temporal arteritis

What to do:

Psychogenic
- ○ reassure
- ○ simple analgesics and tranquillizers not much help
- ○ is it a sign of depression? – tricyclics might help
- ○ social manipulation

Migraine
- ○ prophylaxis – clonidine, pizotifen, propranolol
- ○ ergot compounds
- ○ analgesics
- ○ metoclopramide
- ○ rest in darkened room
- ○ referral to migraine clinic

Raised intracranial pressure and meningitis
- ○ hospital admission

Post-traumatic
- ○ rest, sedation
- ○ convalescence must be gradual after head injury

Extracranial
- ○ specific treatment, e.g. steroids for temporal arteritis

Non-accidental Injury

What might it be:

8000 cases of non-accidental injury reported each year in England. Over 100 deaths annually.

In a suspected case, consider also:
- accidental injury
- a bleeding diathesis
- osteogenesis imperfecta
- skin infections
- birth injury

Assessment:

History
- previous frequent attendances at surgery
- recurrent minor illnesses
- failure to thrive
- injuries to siblings
- delay between accident occurring and your help being requested
- explanation of injury inadequate
- explanation too plausible
- history of disturbed parental behaviour

Examination
- examine child from head to foot
- keep detailed notes
- make sketches if possible
- note child's general appearance –
    - nutritional status
    - cleanliness
    - apprehensive expression, etc.
- note apparent age of any injuries

Look for
- bruises around mouth, on ears, on chin
- pinch marks on cheeks, body, limbs
- grip marks on body
- bruising on body
- bite marks
- strap marks
- imprints, e.g. hair brush
- burns
    - scalds to hands
    - feet
    - buttocks
    - cigarette burns
- localized swellings
- black eyes
- mouth injuries, e.g. torn frenulum
- bone injuries
- evidence of internal injuries –
    - subdural haematoma
    - ruptured liver, etc
Remember that poisoning may be non-accidental

What is it:
○ relate injuries to child's age – falls and bumps common in toddlers
○ is non-accidental injury likely in view of what you know of the family
○ non-accidental injury commoner when –
    ○ previous accidents have occurred
    ○ there is social stress, e.g. housing problems
    ○ there is marital stress
    ○ parents are of low intelligence, alcoholic, of violent propensity, etc.
    ○ child is a result of unwanted pregnancy
    ○ mother is aged under 20
    ○ parents were themselves battered
    ○ there is isolation from the extended family
    ○ mother–infant bonding was deficient

Children particularly at risk are –
    ○ youngest or first-born
    ○ premature infants
    ○ illegitimate children
    ○ 'difficult' children
    ○ children in foster homes
    ○ mentally or physically handicapped
    ○ female children in certain ethnic groups

What to do:
○ ensure child's safety
○ admit to hospital
○ inform admitting doctor of your suspicions
○ if lack of parental co-operation, child can be removed from home through Place of Safety Order (arranged by Social Services Dept and NSPCC).
○ inform Social Services Dept of your suspicions in any case

Follow-up
○ attend case conference
○ note results of investigations carried out in hospital
○ on-going support for family

Psychiatric (see also Section D)

What might it be:
○ Acute emotional disturbance due to domestic or social crisis or bereavement
○ Depression
○ Anxiety
○ Hypomania
○ Psychosis
○ Dementia

Assessment:

History
- Premorbid personality
- Previous history of mental illness
- Recent state of mind
- Social/domestic situation
- Alcohol/drugs
- Other relevant information, e.g. recent confinement

Examination
- Overall appearance
- Communication
- Affect
- Level of agitation/depression
- Thought processes – evidence of psychosis
- Contact with reality
- Evidence of drug taking or alcohol
- Risk of suicide
- Evidence of confusion
- Degree of aggression
- Relationship/attitude to others

What is it:

○ **Emotional crisis in reaction to situation**
- Behaviour may seem out of proportion to immediate precipitating cause especially if underlying marital stress or exhaustion
- The individual presented as the patient may not be the one most in need of help, e.g. hysterical wife of alcoholic husband
- Common in adolescents, married women, at weekends and Bank Holidays

○ **Anxiety or depressive neurosis**
- usually a history of previous problems
- may be a thinly disguised attempt to get more drugs
- suicide a possible risk especially in the bereaved and those with no close family

○ **Manic-depressive illness**
- hypomania builds up over several weeks intense energy and drive and low sleep requirements, ending in exhaustion
- history of manic-depressive personality
- suicide a real danger

○ **Acute psychosis**
- difficulty in establishing rapport
- evidence of paranoid or other delusion; hallucinations
- bizarre behaviour
- thought block can sometimes be demonstrated

                    – may result from taking LSD

○ **Dementia**
- usually elderly
- usually history of deterioration
- may be agitated and/or depressed or frightened
- distant memory may be retained
- recent memory lost

○ **Organic dementias and psychoses include**
- hypothyroidism
- megaloblastic anaemia
- uraemia
- cerebral tumours
- poisoning
- head injury

What to do:

○ **Domestic crisis**
- try not to get involved
- beware of taking sides
- keep calm
- listen and reassure
- avoid providing or prescribing drugs: they can become the family's way of handling every crisis
- advise counsellor if indicated

○ **Anxiety or depressive neurosis**
- management is a long term matter
- in an emergency, the patient can usually be comforted and reassured that he or she will recover in time
- short term tranquillizers (maximum 3 days) may be needed for severe anxiety
- the family also need explanation and reassurance
- admission to hospital rarely needed

○ **Manic-depressive illness**
- adjust drugs if already being prescribed – may have stopped taking maintenance therapy
- seek admission to hospital if severe hypomania or suicidal risk
- remember treatment started *de novo* will take a long time to take effect
- support family

○ **Acute psychosis**
As for manic-depressive illness but also
- assess risks to others and seek admission under Section 4 if necessary.

○ **Dementia**
- listen and reassure both patient and relatives
- drugs unhelpful and likely to make matters worse

○ **Urgent sedation of violent patient**
- Diazepam 10–20 mg i.m. or i.v.
- Chlorpromazine 25–100 mg i.m.

The Mental Health Act 1983 – application for compulsory admission

○ Only the nearest relative or an approved social worker can make an application.

○ The nearest relative is
husband or wife,
son or daughter,
father or mother,
brother or sister,
grandparent, grandchild,
uncle or aunt,
nephew or niece.

N.B. 1. The relative with whom the patient 'ordinarily resides' or from whom care is received is held to be the nearest.
2. A person with whom an unmarried, deserted or separated patient has been living for at least 5 years is deemed to be a relative.

○ An approved social worker must:
have undergone specialized training;

make an application 'as soon as practicable' if asked to by the nearest relative;

interview the patient before making an application or see the patient after, if the patient has been detained in hospital by an application from the nearest relative.

○ **Section 4 (Emergency admission for assessment)**
Applied for by an approved social worker for the nearest relative

Supported by medical recommendation made by one doctor who, if practicable, should have previous knowledge of the patient

Applicant and doctor must have seen the patient in the last 24 hours

Patient must be admitted within 24 hours, or earlier, of application or medical recommendation

Duration of 72 hours

N.B. Admission must be 'urgently necessary'

○ **Section 2 (Admission for assessment)**
Applied for by an approved social worker or nearest relative

Supported by medical recommendations from two doctors including one approved under s.12 and, if practicable, one with knowledge of the patient

Maximum time allowed between examination by the two doctors is 5 days

Duration of 28 days

Patient has right to a Mental Health Review Tribunal in the first 14 days

Copies of the medical recommendations forms are carried by approved social workers. They may also be obtained free of charge from
DHSS Store,
Health Publications Unit,
No. 2 Site,
Manchester Road,
Heywood,
Lancashire, OL10 2PZ.

Sexual Assault

What might it be:

Rape
Unlawful sexual intercourse with a woman by force and against her will. 'Intercourse' here constitutes any degree of penetration, from entry of tip of penis between labia majora to full penetration into vagina, with or without emission of seminal fluid.

Intercourse with children
Intercourse with a girl under the age of 16 years is illegal, even if consent is given.

Intercourse with mental defectives
It is an offence for a man to have intercourse with a woman who is classified as being mentally subnormal or severely abnormal.

Incest
It is an offence for a man to have intercourse with his granddaughter, daughter, sister, half-sister or mother.

A woman may not have intercourse with her grandson, son, brother, half-brother or father.

Indecent assault
May be committed by either a man or a woman.

Range of possible acts very wide.

Assessment:

The person you are most likely to be required to examine is alleged victim of sexual offence.

The person is likely to be emotionally disturbed; many reactions are observed from withdrawal into stunned silence to hysteria.

Great care is needed in handling this.

Always have a chaperone.

Aim is to determine whether intercourse has taken place and to note any injuries, not to act as judge.

Examination must be conducted in surgery or hospital. Consent required from victim or parents/guardians if under 16.

History
○ place of incident
○ course of events
○ resistance used
○ loss of consciousness
○ menstruating

Examination
○ general appearance
○ distressed
○ dishevelled
○ clothes
    ○ stains
    ○ tears, etc.
    retain for forensic examination
○ examine whole body for injuries

Look for
O bruises and abrasions, particularly on thighs, arms, back, face and neck
O bites or suction marks on breast or neck
O bitten nipples

Genitalia
O pubic hair
    O matting by semen
    O comb for foreign hairs
    O pluck sample for forensic examination
O vulva – bruising, swelling, etc.
O hymen – fresh tears
O vaginal – bruising, swelling, laceration

Samples
O vaginal fluid for spermatozoa
O swabs for sexually transmitted disease
O pubic hair (*see above*)
O blood for grouping

Keep copious notes.

What to do:

O Comfort and reassure
O Refer to counsellor, Rape Crisis centre or local women's aid group if appropriate
O Consider safety of child who appears to be victim of incest

(N.B.   Once reported to a Social Worker, the police have to be involved.)

Sore Throat

What might it be:
○ At least 60% are viral even in children with obvious tonsillitis – some are glandular fever
○ In adults without tonsillitis, the proportion due to viral infection is probably much higher
(Beware of acute leukaemia)

Assessment:
○ General condition – is the patient toxic and ill?
○ Local condition – are the tonsils and cervical lymph nodes massively enlarged; is there possibility of peritonsillar abscess?
○ Investigation: not usually helpful
　– Throat swab may show pathogenic bacteria
　– Full blood count may show lymphocytosis, suggesting virus infection or polymorphonuclear leukocytosis, suggesting bacterial infection
　– Paul–Bunnell test in glandular fever may not be positive until third week of illness

What is it:
○ Viral infection –most likely
○ Bacterial infection – a proportion
○ Suspect peritonsillar abscess in someone with several days' history, severe unilateral pain, difficulty in swallowing, trismus and massive tonsillar swelling worse on one side than the other

What to do:
○ Inform, reassure, advise probable course
○ Fluids plus aspirin or paracetamol
○ No evidence antibiotics help but most doctors give penicillin V if patient ill, tonsils large and purulent and cervical glands enlarged or if scarletinaform rash
○ Do not give ampicillin. It causes a rash with glandular fever
○ Routine throat swabs are not necessary but may be helpful in recurring tonsillitis
○ Full blood count and Paul–Bunnell are useful if the course is prolonged beyond 2 weeks.
○ Peritonsillar abscess – admit to hospital. If unavoidable delay, give benzylpenicillin, 1 megaunit i.m.

Stroke

What might it be:

○ Cerebrovascular accident with brain damage due to:
- haemorrhage
- thrombosis
- embolus

○ Predisposing factors:
- old age
- atherosclerosis
- hypertension
- obesity, inactivity
- smoking
- cardiac abnormalities causing emboli, e.g. mitral valve disease, ventricular aneurysm
- drugs, e.g. oral contraceptive in smokers and older women
- diabetes

○ Rare possibilities:
- cerebral tumour, chronic subdural haematoma, cerebral abscess.

Assessment:

History
- Age
- Predisposing factors
- Is condition stable or worsening
- Symptoms

Examination
- Level of consciousness (*see also* below, p. 163, The Unconscious Patient)
- Central nervous system signs – always unilateral

What is it:

Thrombosis
- most likely
- acute onset but picture evolves over a few hours
- often at night

Haemorrhage
- rapid onset
- often during exertion
- signs develop over course of few minutes
- likely to be associated with hypertension

(**N.B.** Subarachnoid haemorrhage occurs in younger age group, associated with severe headache; like a blow on the back of the head, and meningism)

Embolism
- most rapid onset
- sudden development of signs
- evidence of source

What to do: ○ Unconscious patient – *see* next subsection
○ Severely disabled:
   ○ Admit to hospital if
      – home care is inadequate
      – family wish it
   ○ Care at home if
      – relatives can cope
      – community nursing care available
      – patient wishes it
○ Mildly disabled:
   ○ Care at home unless unable to cope.
      – nursing care and mobilization
      watch for faecal impaction/retention with overflow
      pressure sores
      contractures
      – treat hypertension *carefully*

The Unconscious Patient

What might it be:

Neurological
- O cerebrovascular accident
- O cerebral tumour
- O head injury
- O meningitis
- O epilepsy

Metabolic
- O hypoglycaemia
- O ketoacidosis
- O uraemia
- O hepatic failure
- O adrenal failure
- O hypothyroidism

Other
- O terminal event
- O hypothermia
- O poisoning – drugs, alcohol
- O hysteria

Assessment:

History
- O try to obtain a history from neighbours or relatives if possible
- O is the patient known to be diabetic/hypertensive/epileptic, etc.
- O has he or she been on any medication
- O has the patient complained of any symptoms, e.g. headache, vomiting, recently
- O has his or her recent behaviour been normal
- O has there been any recent injury or accident
- O was the onset of unconsciousness sudden

Examination
- O examine the situation in which the patient was found
- O look for pill bottles, suicide notes, alcohol, signs of disturbance or attack
- O examine the patient
  - Medic/Alert bracelet
  - obvious injury/haemorrhage
  - colour and temperature of skin
  - any venepuncture marks
  - smell on breath – ketones, alcohol, hepatic foetor
  - is breathing normal in depth and pattern
  - rate and rhythm of pulse
  - any incontinence
  - take temperature with low reading thermometer.
- O make a routine examination of the systems, paying particular attention to:
  - blood pressure
  - heart rate, rhythm and sounds
  - peripheral pulses, carotid bruit
  - state of hydration
  - pupils and fundi
  - neck stiffness
  - evidence of focal neurological lesion
  - jaundice, cyanosis, etc.
  - stigmata of liver disease

What is it:

Cerebrovascular accident
○ sudden onset
○ past history, e.g. hypertension
○ evidence of hypertension, atherosclerosis, source of emboli
○ focal neurological deficit
○ head turned away from side of hemiplegia
○ Cheyne–Stokes respiration
○ cyanosis

Cerebral tumour
○ gradual onset
○ papilloedema
○ focal neurological signs
○ raised blood pressure
○ slow pulse
○ probably recent history of illness/behavioural disturbance

Meningitis
○ gradual onset
○ pyrexia
○ signs of meningeal irritation
○ short history of malaise, headache, etc.

Head injury
○ sudden onset
○ obvious injury
○ pallor
○ may be bradycardia, diminished reflexes
○ if intracranial haemorrhage – focal neurological signs, ipsilateral dilated pupil

Epilepsy
○ sudden onset
○ known history
○ evidence of injury, tongue-biting, etc.
○ urinary incontinence

Hypoglycaemia
○ sudden onset
○ known diabetic on treatment
○ sweating
○ shallow respiration
○ pulse and BP normal
○ may be incontinence of urine
○ if urine available for testing it will show no ketones (may show sugar if urine has been in bladder for some time)

Ketoacidosis
○ gradual onset
○ history of vomiting, malaise, etc.
○ dehydration
○ low blood pressure
○ deep sighing (kussmaul respiration)
○ weak pulse
○ ketones and sugar in urine

Uraemia
○ gradual onset
○ probably known history of renal disease
○ signs of hypovolaemia or fluid overload
○ acute cardiac failure

Hepatic failure
○ gradual onset
○ jaundice – usually not marked
○ liver may be palpable
○ other stigmata of liver disease – spider naevi, purpura, palmar erythema, etc.
○ hepatic foetor

Adrenal failure
○ usually acute on chronic onset
○ hyperpigmentation
○ hypotension
○ recent history of malaise, gastrointestinal disturbance

Hypothyroidism
○ gradual onset
○ low temperature
○ stigmata of the disease – pale, dry skin; coarse thin hair; myxoedema, etc.

Hypothermia
○ gradual onset
○ rectal temperature below 35 °C
○ may be evidence of injury, e.g. fractured hip
○ may be stigmata of hypothyroidism (see above)

Poisoning
○ sudden onset
○ suicide note
○ pills or bottles
○ venepuncture marks
○ alcohol – bottles in evidence, smell on breath
○ signs of specific poisons, e.g.
   – cherry-red colour in carbon monoxide poisoning
   – respiratory depression and blistering of skin in barbiturate poisoning, etc.

Hysteria
○ sudden onset
○ history of mental/behavioural disturbance
○ absence of physical signs

What to do:
○ in all unconscious patients – ensure patent airway, place in coma position, keep warm but not overheated
○ if hypoglycaemia is suspected – give i.v. glucose or glucagon
○ if patient remains unconscious, admit urgently to hospital unless firm diagnosis of hysteria can be made, or this is an expected event in a terminal illness
○ comfort relatives and inform as much as possible

Vascular

What might it be: Nearly all acute vascular problems in the peripheral circulation affect the lower limbs predominantly.

○ Venous
  - DVT in pelvic or leg pains, associated with bed rest, varicose veins, cardiac failure, dehydration, neoplasia, surgery, pregnancy, oral contraception

○ Arterial
  - Thrombosis in atheromatous artery
  - Embolism from left atrium (atrial fibrillation, mitral stenosis) or left ventricle (myocardial infarction)

Assessment: ○ Deep vein thrombosis (DVT)
  - may be silent and present with acute complications
    e.g. pulmonary embolus or chronic complications, e.g. postphlebitic leg
  - when apparent
    - discomfort, discolouration, swelling of leg or foot
    - skin shiny and warm
    - dilated superficial veins
    - positive Homan's sign

○ Arterial
  - sudden severe pain in leg
  - skin cold and pale
  - no pulses beyond occlusion
  - loss of power
  - loss of sensation

What to do: ○ DVT
  - anticoagulants (heparin + warfarin)
  - admit to hospital

○ Arterial
  - pain relief (morphine)
  - expose and cool affected leg
  - heparin
  - admit to hospital (vascular unit)

Vertigo

What might it be: There is considerable confusion over the clinical definition of vertigo because of uncertainty about the nature and causes.

In general practice types are –

	%
Epidemic vertigo + benign positional vertigo (vestibular neuronitis)	80 (5–6 cases per year)
Méniére's syndrome	15 (1–2 cases per year)
Mini-strokes	3 (1 every 2 years)
Chronic otitis media	1 (1 every 5-10 years)
Others, e.g. acute infection, trauma, multiple sclerosis	1
	100

Assessment:

General examination
○ TPR
○ BP

Ears
○ normal
○ chronic otitis media
○ hearing

CNS
○ nystagmus
○ reflexes
○ power and movement

What is it:

Epidemic vertigo
○ went to bed well
○ on awakening in morning
    ○ sensation of rotation on moving head
    ○ falls on standing
    ○ nausea and vomiting
    ○ victim usually lies still in bed with eyes shut
    ○ vertigo worse on moving head
    ○ nystagmus may be present
    ○ no other abnormal signs
    ○ attack passes within few days
    ○ return of vertigo on sudden movements, (e.g. looking up, on getting up and going to bed)
    ○ recurrent attacks not uncommon (may be benign positional vertigo)
    ○ cause unknown (no evidence that it is an infection)
    ○ young and middle-aged adults affected.

Ménière's syndrome
○ cause unknown
○ pathology said to be −
    ○ dilatation membraneous labyrinth
    ○ destruction of sensory cells in cochlea and ampulla
    ○ middle-aged adults
    ○ attacks (few hours − days) −
        ○ vertigo
        ○ nausea and vomiting
        ○ tinnitus
        ○ deafness (may become permanent)

What to do:

Make a diagnosis!
○ most likely are epidemic vertigo or benign positional vertigo
○ no specific therapy available
○ general measures
    ○ reassure + + that **not** due to −
        ○ tumours
        ○ blood pressure
        ○ strokes
○ explain nature and course
○ avoid sudden quick movements
○ possible relief with promethazine, prochlorperazine.

Section D

PSYCHIATRY IN GENERAL PRACTICE

Psychiatry in General Practice

In practice it is important to distinguish –

○ distress in a normal mind:
  unhappiness──▶depression
  fear──────────▶phobias
  anxiety────────▶agitation
  excitement──▶hypomania, etc.

○ distress in a disordered mind:
  schizophrenia and allied conditions
  manic depressive psychosis

○ distress in a diseased mind:
  dementia
  confusional states

○ distress in a poisoned mind:
  drug ⎫ ⎧ abuse/access
  or   ⎬ ⎨ or
  alcohol ⎭ ⎩ withdrawal

○ distress associated with
  fear or presence of
  physical illness:
  anxiety and depression might
  be considered normal
  experiences when facing life's
  stresses, especially illness.

  ○ most patients will, therefore, suffer distress and
  ○ most will not require specific psychiatric medication provided that
  ○ most are given acknowledgement of their state of mind, and the
    opportunity to ventilate it.

Problems may become large when the patient (and enormous when the doctor) fails to acknowledge this distress.

Concepts

○ mental disorders are as diverse as the individuals who suffer them.
○ classification may only be made by intentionally ignoring this individuality.
○ there is no clear cut division between the mind and the body either in the genesis or the expression of illness.
○ constantly re-educating ourselves and our patients about these concepts may be our most effective therapy.

Attention

Observe every aspect of the patient's behaviour–
○ how he enters the room
○ who he comes with and who he leaves behind
○ where and how he sits
○ the words he uses as well as what he says
○ how he is dressed
○ unusual smells, viz, alcohol or halitosis
○ acknowledge (to yourself) what you feel about the patient,
  i.e. does he annoy me, depress me
○ pay attention to what the patient says.

Facts

In a hypothetical practice of 2500 we may find (RCGP (1983). *Present State and Future Needs* 6th edn. (Lancaster: MTP Press))

Acute major disorders	Cases per annum
Neurotic disorders	300
Chronic mental illness	55
Severe depression	12
Severe mental handicap	10
Suicide attempts	4
Completed suicide	1 every 3 years

Social pathology	
Chronic alcoholism (known cases)	5
Alcoholism probably unknown to GP	25
Juvenile delinquency	5–7
'Problem' families	5–10
One-parent families with children under 15	60

Referral rates to psychiatrists vary enormously from survey to survey, from 17.7 to 160.6 per 10000 at risk.

Strategies for management

○ consider − 'the doctor as drug' and
     'the doctor as dangerous drug'

○ collaboration with
  ○ other members of practice staff
  ○ other patients or patients' groups
  ○ local groups and agencies
  on the principle 'when the going gets tough learn to enjoy it or get someone else to lend a hand'

○ pre-emption of crises − adolescence, bereavement
○ knowledge of people at risk
○ open access wherever possible.

Anxiety

Anxiety is a necessary and normal part of healthy life. The patient presents because it is unpleasant, not because it is abnormal.

In the consulting room it may be seen
○ when there is a fear of illness
○ in established physical or mental illness
○ recurrently or persistently in the 'worrying type'
○ in tension states
○ secondary to an underlying mental illness

The physiology of 'fright and fight' is normal but variable
○ depends on personality, age and experience, precise location and company, culture and concomitant drug therapy or abuse

'*Neuroses*' in the broadest sense form over 60% of the GP's workload.

It may be helpful to divide between–
○ simple anxiety
○ anxiety states and tension states
○ depression
○ obsessional neuroses and phobias
○ all these may be mixed and interwoven, and change with time.

Symptom peaks

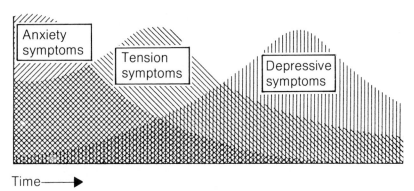

Time———▶

Simple anxiety

This is the fear (usually of disease) engendered by an experience in a normal person.

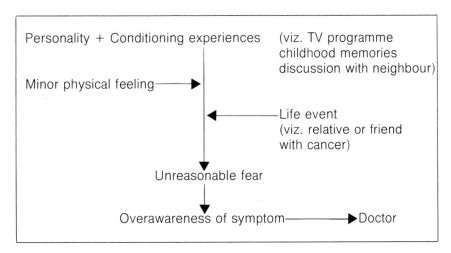

Presentation may be influenced by what other people have said to patient, or by the advice he has sought – 'the lay referral system'.

Conditioning experience or life event may be the most significant point to discover, to enable doctor to understand patient's reason for presentation.

If a symptom remains unexplained, it may be necessary to check on–
O previous experience of illness, personal or second-hand.
O the diseases currently and in the past, experienced by his family or close friends.
O his beliefs about physical functions, including cultural beliefs.
O symbolism of the symptom to the patient.
O recent life events, anniversaries, dreams.
O recent change in life circumstances or 'passage'.

Ask yourself 'Why did the patient come, what did the patient want?'

Ask the patient 'What is it that you are worried is the matter with you?'

Reassurance can only follow if these factors are uncovered, and once suitable steps have been taken, telling the patient not only what he has got, but also what he has **not** got. Give accurate and simple explanations. Know common causes of misunderstanding. Listen carefully. Performing an examination is often in itself therapeutic.

Failed reassurance is indicated by continued questioning, unhappiness, repeated consultations, often with a relative, or suggestion of further action or investigation. Early detection of failure to reassure is important if persistent symptoms or unnecessary investigation are to be avoided.

'Irritation and asperity shown by the doctor under pressure of work are probably the biggest single cause of failure to reassure.' (Keith Hodgkin)

Anxiety and tension

A state of pure extreme anxiety is rare clinically and what is often put under this heading is usually a result of more longstanding tension or personality factors.

Presentation
O restlessness, frustration, unhappiness, depression, weariness
O disturbed concentration, irritability, nervousness
O excessive sentimentality and loss of emotional control
O decreased appetite and weight loss
O sleeplessness, troubled dreams
O exhaustion, often in spite of sleep
O somatic sensations
      O headaches, dizziness, blackouts
      O weakness, butterflies
      O breathlessness, overbreathing, air swallowing and flatulence
      O increased micturition
      O disturbed bowel function
      O palpitations, nausea

Signs are those of
O adrenergic overactivity
O body language ⎫
O surgery behaviour ⎬ indicating stress
O frequent attendance

Source of stress must be sought, but may sometimes be obtained more easily by observation, open ended questions or intuition when conventional 'history taking' techniques fail.

Explore
O areas of conflict or frustration
O relationships at work and with family
O previous behaviour
O culmination of small stresses
O sudden removal of stress with latent period

Diagnosis may be aided by –
O good knowledge of local events and family events
O reducing anxiety levels by
    O attitudes of staff
    O attitudes of doctor
    O surgery or waiting room surroundings
O using paramedical help (health visitors, receptionists)
O using counselling methods, if appropriate
O 'flash' technique
O observing **patient** at all times, especially during examination.

Treatment
O ventilation may be enough
O adequate reassurance
O allowing patient to express his expectations for treatment
O doctor as drug first
O tranquillizers last
O avoid
    O barbiturates
    O tranquillizers in long term, with repeat prescription
    O prescribing if dependence a major hazard

O consider
    O depression and antidepressants
    O β-blockers
    O displacement activity
    O counselling sessions – with other agencies if necessary
    O group work   } as future aims
    O relaxation therapy }

Differential diagnosis of anxiety in various forms:

Diagnosis	Suggested by	Confirmed by
Depression	*see page* 177	
Dementia	Disorientation in time, place and person	
Psychotic states	Psychotic symptoms	
Thyrotoxicosis	Physical signs of hyperthyroidism	Thyroid function tests
Hypercalcaemia	Cancer with bony secondaries (Hyperparathyroidism)	Calcium levels taken without a cuff
CO_2 narcosis	Chronic obstructive airways disease Cyanosis, bounding large volume pulse	Blood gases
Alcohol withdrawal	History, including early morning vomiting, recurrent absence from work, symptoms of delirium tremens	Signs of liver disease Disturbed liver tests Alcohol levels
Hypoglycaemia	Usually insulin-dependent diabetic	Blood sugar
Overuse or abuse of stimulant drug	i.e. amphetamines salbutamol	Urine tests or therapeutic withdrawal

Serious organic disease, where fear is predominant and has masked the presentation of more 'important' diagnostic symptoms or signs.

Depression (Affective Illness)

Depression encompasses inappropriate sadness and low mood state. The problem is in distinguishing between **normal** and **marked** depression.

Most persons faced with a physical or mental illness will be anxious or depressed. Though this may be normal in degree, it may alter the presentation and course of the illness and must always be dealt with in management.

Clinical picture

Endogenous depression	Reactive depression
Mood variation slight	Varying from day to day
Worst in mornings	Worst when tired
Complaints unchanged and persistent	Varying complaints
Reassurance no help	Reassurance helps
Obsessed	Distractible
Behaviour underlines statements	Behaviour often belies statements
Retarded and slow	May be overactive and anxious
Concentration poor ⎫ interference with normal life Habits change ⎭	May not interfere with normal life
Libido lost	Faulty sexual relationships may precede illness
Suicide likely	Suicide in word but not deed
Wakes early, very tired	Difficulty getting to sleep or sleeps long and wakes tired

There may be a mixture of symptoms.

Significance

Prevalence: 50 per 2500 per year (12 of these will be severe).

Age: more commonly recognized in second half of life, but it is probable that much childhood and adolescent depression goes unrecognized.

NOTE:
○ the separation reactions of childhood
○ identity crises of adolescence
○ stealing in children, adolescents and middle-aged women
○ sexual deviations in middle-aged men
○ alcoholism
○ confusion and bodily obsessions in old age

There may be **sexual, class and cultural differences** in symptom presentations:

Western women:	palpitations, nausea, crying (F>M in West)
Asian men:	fears and loss of potency (M>F in India)
West Indian men:	fear of loss of strength and inability to work
Middle class:	loneliness and guilt
Working class:	powerlessness, hopelessness

Risk factors

- over 30
- loss of mother before 11
- more than three children under 14 years old at home
- no job
- no outside interest
- low income group
- no extended family
- no close confidante
- poor communication with spouse
- loss of close relative or friend within 2 years
- low self-esteem

Severe depression

- loss of energy, decrease in activity
- loss of sexual drive
- sleep disturbance
- constipation
- loss of weight, or abnormal gain
- headache
- amenorrhoea
- abnormal pains
- loss of diurnal variation in mood and function
- hallucinations
- inability to cope
- retardation
- perplexity
- preoccupation with own symptoms
- self depreciation
- ideas of reference
- delusion of guilt
- hypochondriacal
- facies and position of hands
- watery eyes, red eyes
- signs of abnormal alcohol intake
- anger

Triggers

- behavioural or life events
  - loss or threatened loss of spouse, house, pet, job, prestige
  - small event as 'last straw'
  - sometime (3 weeks–2 years) after: 'after the ball is over'.

- during a 'passage' or change in life
  - puerperium
  - retirement
  - engagement or marriage
  - move

- symbolically, associated with
  - anniversary of tragic event (viz. death of spouse, etc.)
  - entering a new decade ('life begins at forty')

- physical illness, associated with
  - virus infections, (viz. influenza,) glandular fever
  - organic neurology, (viz. head injury,) stroke, Parkinsonism, dementia

- otherwise symptomless carcinoma, especially of lung, tuberculosis
- hypothyroidism
- anaemia, especially Vit. B12 or folate deficiency
- hypercalcaemia (often with anxiety)
- menopause
- premenstrual tension
- surgical operation, especially hysterectomy

○ drug effects or withdrawal, viz.
- contraceptive pill
- tranquillizers and sleeping tablets
- methyl dopa, reserpine and other hypotensives
- steroids
- stopping amphetamines or appetite depressants

○ life styles, associated with
- isolation
- alcoholism
- institutional living
- cultural inhibition of aggression

○ early stages of
- schizophrenia
- dementia

Management of depression

> 'Could this be depression?'
> 'Can it be helped by me?'
> 'Is there a risk of suicide?'

○ assess suicide risk, hospitalization if necessary.
○ assess precipitating factors – how can they be altered?
○ PAY ATTENTION
○ allow ventilation of grief, guilt, anger, etc.
○ investigate possible underlying physical causes
○ deal sympathetically with symptoms and fear of physical illness.

Drugs

○ **Tricyclic antidepressants:**
 ○ small supplies on each prescription but give effective doses in severe depression.
 ○ see patient regularly: increase dose gradually.
 ○ if sleep disturbance, consider main dose at night e.g. amitriptyline 25mg t.d.s. and 75mg nocte
 ○ warn about time before drugs work
 ○ warn about side effects
 ○ taper off slowly after 3-4 months

○ **Monoamine oxidase inhibitors** if strong reactive element.
 Use with caution and full understanding of the side effects and interactions.

○ **Electroconvulsive therapy** if refractive.
 Consider side effects and patient's and relatives' attitudes carefully.

Suicide

○ reporting varies from country to country
○ 4300 per year in UK (1 per GP every 3 years)
○ 15% of psychotic depressives will kill themselves
○ seasonal incidence – high in spring and late summer

Vulnerables
○ men over 70
○ women over 60
○ urban
○ single
○ childless
○ isolated
○ unemployed
○ Protestant or irreligious
○ recently widowed or divorced
○ family history of suicide
○ past history of suicide attempt
○ beginning and end of depressive illness
○ agitation, guilt, inadequacy
○ alcohol +
○ access to method
○ 70% communicate their intentions to someone
○ 40% do so by explicit statement to someone
○ 40% visit their GP in week before they die
○ 70% visit their GP in 3 months before they die
○ many use the medication prescribed in these consultations

Attempted suicide

Other names – parasuicide, suicidal gestures, uncompleted suicide.

For every successful suicide 20 make the gesture.

Sometimes an obvious gesture misfires and results in death.
Attendances at Casualty Departments and admissions to Medical Wards dealing with self-imposed poisoning bear witness to the dramatic increase in this behaviour in the UK.

Methods often seem to follow a 'fashion' or suicide of public figure.
○ 40% have past history of attempts
○ 20% will repeat within a year

	Attempted suicide	Suicide
Incidence	Rising dramatically	Steady or declining
Sex	Women>men	Men>women
Age	Younger	Late middle age
Social class	Lower	Upper
Childhood	Broken home	Bereavement
Physical health	Good	Often a terminal illness or handicap
Personality	Poorly adjusted	Often well adjusted
Alcohol	Often drinking before attempt	Alcoholism
Background	Situational illness	Depressive
Precipitation	Acute personal crisis	Guilt, hopelessness, painful or disabling illness
Setting	Impulsive but with forewarning and in presence of others	Carefully planned Giving warning but carried out alone
Methods	Multiple drug self-poisoning or wrist cutting	Massive effective single drug use. Violent methods, e.g. guns or hanging

Pointers for GP:
○ open access in crisis even with appointment system.
○ out of hours service.
○ great care in all prescribing, especially psychotropics.
○ establishing and using personal relationship to forestall attempt, prevent crisis if attempt made, and prevent pattern of recurrent attempts being established by arranging suitable help, regular 'ventilation' or psychotherapy.
○ in the very disturbed personality, avoid being trapped into response to manipulative threat, by creating a contract, i.e. constructive responses to stress . . . . rather than reverse.
○ keep in contact with elderly bereaved, etc., who may be at special risk: ancilliary staff very important here.

Manic depressive (or bipolar) illness

Classically, cyclothymic personality, pyknic physique, family history.

Hypomanic or manic phase alternates with depressed phase – the former is more damaging and difficult to deal with. Recurrent episodes. Attack lasts 3–6 weeks.

Signs
○ self assertion   ○ overspending   ○ elation
○ extravagance   ○ religious obsession   ○ pressure of speech

- unduly secretive
- irritability
- sexual disinhibition
- campaigns
- flights of ideas
- grandiose ideas
- violence if restrained
- rejection of suggestion of mental illness

Management
- use bargaining or symptoms of physical illness to gain patient's acceptance of hospital admission, if possible.
- if not, suggest removal from emotionally charged atmosphere + drugs: haloperidol 1.5–10 mg t.d.s. or chlorpromazine. May need police powers (section 136) or section 29.
- long term lithium: 800–1600 mg daily initially, reducing to 400–800 daily as maintenance. Control with serum estimation. Use psychiatric backup where possible. May need antidepressants during depressed phase. Side effects: cardiac arrhythmias, renal damage, thyroid damage, excessive weight gain, acute reversible dementia.
  Signs of lithium toxicity: anorexia, coarse tremor, diarrhoea and vomiting, thirst.

Organic Psychoses

What are they: Major mental disorders of unknown cause, hence their classification has to be descriptive and their management pragmatic.

Classification

- senile and presenile dementias
- alcoholic psychoses
- drug psychoses
- schizophrenic psychoses
- manic-depressive psychoses
- paranoid states

Clinical features

There are no absolutely clear clinical divisions between these disorders. There are some common features:
- mood disturbances
- delusions and hallucinations
- thought disturbances
- paranoid feelings

but there is predominance of some features among these syndromes

- **dementias** – deficiencies of memory and intellect, with bouts of confusion, depression and agitation
- **alcoholic and drug psychoses** produce a variety of clinical features depending on the drugs
- **schizophrenia** – thought derangements, hallucinations, delusions, abnormal affective behaviour, paranoid beliefs, social degeneration
- **manic-depression** – bouts of severe depression and/or mania and hypomania. Often return to normality between episodes.
- some **paranoid states** do not fit other categories, with delusions of self-reference such as persecution, grandeur, litigation, jealousy, love, hate, honour and others.

Significance

- Cause major distress and disturbance to all involved – patient, family, GP and specialist.

- Apart from **alcoholic and drug psychoses** which can be 'cured', the prognosis in dementia, schizophrenia, manic-depression and paranoia is not good.

- **Senile and presenile dementias** are progressive.

- In **schizophrenia** –
    - one third have a single major episode
    - one third suffer recurring attacks with intervening periods of relative normality
    - one third are chronic with persisting symptoms.

- **Manic-depression** tends to be a recurring condition, with normality between attacks.

Assessment

- There are specific tests or investigations to confirm the diagnosis.
- Each patient must be assessed individually and in each attention must be given to –
    - disease process and its effects
    - social circumstances of the patient

○ family situation
○ likely effects of possible therapies including drugs, social help and medical support.

Planned care

○ **Patient** – is he/she able to understand and co-operate in the planned care?

○ **Family** – supportive or rejecting?

○ **Friends** – are there any and what attitudes?

○ **GP**
   ○ having made the diagnosis and decided on lines of treatment–
   ○ is the patient manageable at home?
   ○ can regular support and surveillance be provided by GP or the team?
   ○ consider indications for –
      ○ urgent admission to mental hospital
      ○ referral to psychiatric OPD
      ○ domiciliary visit by specialists.

○ **Specialist**
   ○ decide on type and place of treatment
   ○ arrange regular support and follow-up by community psychiatric services
   ○ possibly admission for short stay or long stay.

Compulsory admission of patient to mental hospital

General points
○ Only use legal compulsion (certification) if voluntary persuasion fails.
○ Unless dramatically urgent arrange for psychiatrist to visit patient at home to try and persuade or to use compulsory procedures.

Mental Health Act 1983
○ **Admission for assessment** (Section 2) (previously section 25 of Mental Health Act of 1959):
   ○ to admit to hospital for 28 days
   ○ two medical practitioners – one an 'approved doctor' (psychiatrist), the other can be GP. Examination must be within 5 days of each other
   ○ application may be made by nearest relative or approved social worker.

○ **Admission for treatment** (Section 3) (previously section 26):
   ○ to admit to hospital for 6 months
   ○ examination by two doctors (one 'approved') within 5 days of each other
   ○ application by nearest relative or approved social worker.

○ **Admission in an emergency** (Section 4) (previously section 29):
   ○ to admit for urgent treatment for 72 hours
   ○ recommendation by one doctor, preferably GP.
   ○ patient must be admitted within 24 hours
   ○ application by nearest relative or approved social worker
   ○ admission to hospital has to be arranged by GP.

Principles of management

General
○ First priority is to organize care and support for the patient by family, friends or sociomedical services.

○ Arrangements must be for long term care.
○ Know the local community services available and learn how to use them.
○ Ensure that someone is in regular contact with patient and family.

Drugs

Antipsychotic drugs are important. They appear to act by interfering with dopaminergic transmission in the brain and may cause parkinsonism and hyperprolactinaemia.

○ Alleviate anxiety
○ Tranquillize
○ Specific antipsychotic effects
○ Antipsychotic drugs will need to be used for long time, regular assessment is necessary to monitor benefits and note side effects
○ Whenever possible only use one drug or as few as possible
○ Antipsychotic drugs are *phenothiazine* derivatives or *lithium*

Self-help from:

○ National Schizophrenia Fellowship,
78/79 Victoria Road,
Surbiton, Surrey KT6 4NS.

○ The Samaritans,
17 Uxbridge Road,
Slough SL1 1SN.
(Branches in local 'phone directories.)

Section E

CLINICAL CARE

Anaemia

What is it

Anaemia is a deficiency of blood haemoglobin level below 12 g per 100 ml.
Anaemia always is secondary to some underlying process.
Anaemia is never a primary 'disease' to be treated *per se*.
Anaemias may be **classified:**
- **defective production of blood cells** due to deficiency of essential factors
- iron deficiency
    - loss through bleeding
    - inadequate intake
    - excessive requirement
- vitamin B_{12}/folic acid (megaloblastic) deficiency
- **excessive blood destruction**
    - haemolysis
        - intrinsic
        - extrinsic.
- **non-production in blood marrow**
    - hypoplastic
        - idiopathic
        - drugs
        - radiation
- **miscellaneous**
    - cancers
    - rheumatoid arthritis
    - kidney/liver diseases
    - hypothyroidism

In general practice more than 90% of anaemias are due to iron deficiency, 9% are megaloblastic and 1% the rest

Significance

- incidence   — 10 per 1000 per annum (25 new cases in a practice of 2500)
- sex distribution   — F : M = 10 : 1 (more common in females++)
- course   — early diagnosis depends on awareness of doctor
- at risk   — infancy
         — women
        - 15 – 50 (menses+)
        - pregnancy
         — food fadists
         — elderly
        - diet
        - underlying disease
         — postgastrectomy

Assessment	Awareness+
	○ is there anaemia?
	    ○ check
	        ○ HB
	        ○ MCV
	        ○ MCHC
	        ○ RBC
	○ underlying cause
	    ○ disease?
	    ○ drugs?
	    ○ diet?

Planned care	○ suspicion index + − cannot rely on appearances ○ diagnosis by blood check ○ definitive treatment as specifically appropriate with iron, hydroxocobalamin or folic acid ○ follow-up ○ long term follow-up and regular assessment is essential to prevent relapse

Cardiac Arrhythmias

What are they
- ○ disturbances of regular activation of ventricles from sinoatrial nodes
- ○ may be benign disorders of faulty conducting mechanism without any cardiac disease
- ○ may be associated with serious heart diseases
- ○ may be caused by non-cardiac disorders such as thyroid diseases, anaemia, excess alcohol or side effects of therapeutic drugs

Clinical features
- ○ there are few specific symptoms or signs apart from the character of the pulse and cardiac auscultation

- ○ **symptoms** may be:
    - ○ palpitations, awareness of heart's action by rate of irregularity
    - ○ intermittent breathlessness
    - ○ intermittent chest pain or discomfort
    - ○ polyuria, associated with tachycardia
    - ○ bouts of dizziness, faintness or syncope

- ○ **signs** may be:
    - ○ character of peripheral pulses
    - ○ cardiac auscultation
    - ○ effects of disturbed circulation as heart failure, hypotension, shock, collapse
    - ○ arterial embolization

Significance
- ○ cardiac arrhythmias are very common
- ○ prognosis depends on type, causation and association with heart disease

Assessment
- ○ possibility of arrhythmias may have to depend on careful history
- ○ examination must include other body systems as well as cardiovascular
- ○ definitive diagnosis requires objective evidence from electrocardiography. A 24 hour or longer tape recording may be necessary
- ○ all but straightforward cases should be assessed by cardiologist

Principles of management
- ○ these depend on the type of arrhythmia

- ○ sinus tachycardia
    - ○ usually symptomless
    - ○ benign, seldom associated with heart disease
    - ○ may occur in anaemia, thyrotoxicosis, alcoholism, fevers or other diseases
    - ○ specific antiarrhythmic therapy is unnecessary

- ○ supraventricular extrasystoles
    - ○ anxiety symptoms
    - ○ rarely associated with cardiac or non-cardiac disease
    - ○ specific therapy: unnecessary, give reassurance and if this does not succeed, then β-blockers may be effective

- ○ supraventricular tachycardias
    - ○ symptoms+
    - ○ may be haemodynamic effects
    - ○ benign usually, but may be result of digitalis toxicity and dangerous in Wolff–Parkinson–White syndrome

- ○ may respond to vagal stimulation manoeuvres
- ○ if persist, refer urgently to hospital where d.c. shock may be used
- ○ prophylaxis with β-blockers or digitalis
- ○ atrial flutter
  - ○ 'sustained' – usually with myocardial disease
  - ○ d.c. shock conversion or digitalization at hospital
  - ○ paroxysmal – often with no heart disease
  - ○ prevent with digitalis or amiodarone
- ○ atrial fibrillation – sustained
  - ○ symptoms+
  - ○ usually with cardiac disease
  - ○ sometimes with non-cardiac disease
  - ○ check for mitral valve disease, hypertension, alcohol + in young, thyroid disease
  - ○ prognosis depends on underlying disease
  - ○ may be benign in elderly
  - ○ digitalis if ventricular rate over 100. Watch for overdosage
  - ○ β-blockers or verapamil may be added if digitilization fails to control rate
  - ○ anticoagulation in mitral valve disease and cardiomyopathy to prevent embolization
- ○ atrial fibrillation – paroxysmal
  - ○ benign usually
  - ○ may become sustained
  - ○ attacks treated with digitalis
  - ○ prophylaxis
    - ○ digitalis
    - ○ disopyramide
    - ○ quinidine
    - ○ amiodarone
  - ○ consider anticoagulation in mitral valve disease and cardiomyopathy
- ○ ventricular extrasystoles
  - ○ usually benign
  - ○ may be associated with myocardial disease
  - ○ specific antiarrhythmic therapy unnecessary
  - ○ note – in susceptible individuals, aggravation by coffee, smoking, tea, alcohol and by digitalis
- ○ ventricular tachycardia
  - ○ usually of serious import, associated with myocardial disease
  - ○ urgent referral to hospital
- ○ sinus bradycardia
  - ○ benign
  - ○ seldom symptomatic
  - ○ note – can be induced by
    - ○ digitalis
    - ○ β-blockers
    - ○ lithium
    - ○ jaundice
    - ○ raised intracranial pressure
    - ○ hypothyroidism

○ **atrioventricular block**
    ○ usually causes severe symptoms from decreased cardiac output
    ○ refer for possible pacemaker therapy

○ **bundle-branch block**
    ○ no symptoms unless complicated by AV block.
    ○ prognostic significance, *minor* if not associated with myocardial disease. *Serious* if underlying myocardial disease or aortic valve disease.
    ○ refer to specialist if symptoms persist.

Chronic Cardiac Failure

What is it
- failure of heart pump
- end result of many possible **causes**
  - coronary artery disease
  - high blood pressure
  - structural defects of heart, congenital and acquired
  - arrhythmias
  - cardiomyopathy
  - lung diseases
  - anaemia
  - thyrotoxicosis

- **left ventricular failure**
  - effort breathlessness
  - paroxysmal nocturnal dyspnoea
  - chest infections
  - basal roles
  - forceful apex beat with displacement
  - third sound gallop

- **right ventricular failure**
  - filling of neck veins
  - breathlessness
  - swelling legs and abdomen
  - large tender liver
  - low urine output
  - weight gain
  - pleural effusion

Significance
- if untreated leads to **death**
- **cure** if cause can be corrected
- **controllable** even if no cure possible
- the earlier the diagnosis the better the outcome

Assessment
- clinical acumen and examination necessary for early diagnosis
- seek out the causes
- helpful investigations in GP
  - e.c.g.
  - chest X-ray
  - blood check
  - urinalysis

Planned care
- patient and family informed of nature of condition
- **GP** initial diagnosis and assessment – refer to specialist if possible remediable conditions or if diagnosis and management are difficult
- **specialist** – referral direct to superspecialist cardiological unit (if one is available) is better than to general physician
- long term care necessary by both GP and specialist

Principles of management
- **rest and exercise** to match cardiac function
- remedy **cause** if possible
- **digitalization** – not only for arrhythmias but also for right ventricular failure – but beware of overdosage
- **diuretics**
- **vasodilators**
- **surgery** to correct defects and improve function

High Blood Pressure

What is it
- ○ diagnosis of high blood pressure is an exercise in mensuration
- ○ levels of over 160/100 on at least three separate occasions for diagnosis (some accept 140/90)
- ○ Over 90% of high blood pressure is primary 'essential' of unknown cause

Possible causes of secondary high blood pressure (less than 10% of cases) CASSIUS
- ○ coarction of aorta (femoral pulses?)
- ○ aldosteronism (Conn's syndrome – Serum K?)
- ○ suprarenal disease (Cushing's syndrome, phaeochromocytoma – appearance history?)
- ○ stenosis of a renal artery (abdominal bruits?)
- ○ inflammation or infection of kidneys (nephritis or pyelonephritis – urine?)
- ○ unilateral kidney disease (urine? serum creatinine?)
- ○ steroids (iatrogenic hypertension), (drug history? pill? liquorice?)

Malignant hypertension (less than 1% of all hypertensives) – very high blood pressure, severe complications and rapid death if untreated

Significance
- ○ incidence
  - – 10–15% of population are hypertensive
  - – 20–30% of adults
  - – 250–375 patients in a practice population of 2500
  - – 6–7 million in UK

- ○ condition of ageing – one half are over 60 when first diagnosed
- ○ sex distribution – F>M
- ○ high blood pressure – a 50% increased risk to life
  - – increased risk of strokes
  - – possible damage to eyes, kidneys and heart
- ○ prognosis related to – age at diagnosis (worse in younger)
  - – sex (worse in males)
  - – level of BP (worse in high BP)
  - – FH (worse when FH of strokes or heart disease)
- ○ effective antihypertensive drugs are available
- ○ early diagnosis of vulnerables is important
  - ○ at risk
    - – males
    - – young (under 60)
    - – high BP
    - – FH+ (CVS – CNS deaths)
    - – Africans and West Indians
    - – diabetics
    - – smokers

Clinical types
- ○ raised BP is the only common sign
- ○ majority have no abnormal symptoms
- ○ majority have no abnormal signs apart from raised BP

Assessment	○ has patient sustained high BP? (take at least three readings on separate days)
	○ is there any underlying cause?
	○ basic investigations?
	    ○ to exclude primary cause?
	    ○ to provide base lines?
	        ○ urinalysis
	        ○ e.c.g.
	        ○ chest X-ray
	        ○ i.v.p.
	        ○ other when indicated
	○ likely prognosis:
	    ○ age?
	    ○ sex
	    ○ BP level
	    ○ FH
	    ○ organ involvement
	    ○ other risk factors

Planned care	**Not all hypertensives need treatment**
	○ think twice with – F>M
	                       – over-60s
	                       – mild BP levels<160/105
	
	Treatment when indicated may be life-long (but not necessarily so)
	○ patient compliance is important
	○ inform and instruct patient
	○ regular review once stabilized: once or twice a year
	○ practice nurse's role in surveillance
	○ in elderly it may be possible to stop therapy without hypertension returning
	
	General (non-drug treatment)
	○ self-help
	○ compliance
	○ weight control
	○ low salt diet
	○ stop smoking
	○ reduce excessive alcohol
	○ stop 'Pill'
	○ correct hyperlipidaemia
	○ more exercise
	
	Practice plan
	○ all adults to have BP checked and recorded every 3–5 years
	○ practice register of hypertensives
	○ regular BP checks and surveillance of those under care
	○ aim to reduce BP below 160/90
	
	Antihypertensives
	○ diuretics
	○ β-blockers
	○ vasodilators
	○ centrally acting antihypertensives
	○ adrenergic neuron blockers
	○ α-adrenoreceptor blockers
	○ ganglion blockers
	○ angiotensin-converting enzyme inhibitors

Ischaemic Heart Disease (IHD)

What is it

○ **IHD** is the result of narrowing of coronary arteries through atherosclerosis (there are other rare causes).

○ **atherosclerosis** of coronary arteries is a local manifestation of a generalized pathological process, hence patients with IHD may also suffer from intermittent claudication, cerebrovascular disease, effects of mesenteric arterial occlusion and others.

○ **clinical effects** depend on extent and speed of occlusion of the coronary arteries, but there is poor correlation between arterial morbid pathologic and clinical syndromes.

○ **clinical effects** may result from damage to –
    ○ myocardium, i.e. infarction, angina, heart failure
    ○ neuromuscular tissues, i.e. dysrhythmias
    ○ endocardium, i.e. thrombus formation and embolization.

○ **causes** are not clear but **risk factors** can be listed –
    ○ sex : higher incidence and poorer prognosis in males
    ○ age : increasing incidence with age, prognosis worse in younger victims
    ○ family history of sudden deaths and heart disease
    ○ raised blood cholesterol and lipids particularly in the familial types in young and middle-aged
    ○ high blood pressure in males under 50
    ○ diabetes
    ○ cigarette smoking
    ○ obesity
    ○ indolence
    ○ possibly stress–tension.

○ **characterized by**
    ○ sudden death
    ○ acute myocardial infarction
    ○ angina (stable and unstable)
    ○ dysrhythmias
    ○ heart failure.

Significance

○ **in UK, one quarter of all deaths** (150 000 per year) are from IHD; it is the largest single cause of death.

○ in a **general practice of 2500** the **annual prevalence** of IHD may be
    ○ deaths – 7 (4 sudden and unexpected)
    ○ acute myocardial infarction – 10
    ○ angina – 20
    ○ heart failure (of all types) – 50
    ○ dysrhythmias – possibly 10.

○ the **natural history** is
    ○ for **acute myocardial infarction:**
        ○ 25% die on first day
        ○ another 10% die in first month
        ○ another 10% die in first year
        ○ another 15% die in 1–5 years
        ○ i.e. 60% dead in 5 years

○ for **angina:**
    ○ 5 year mortality is 25%.

Assessment

○ **clinical presentations**
    ○ sudden unexpected death
    ○ chest pain – persistent (myocardial infarction)
    ○ chest pain – intermittent (angina)
    ○ dysrhythmias
    ○ heart failure (congestive or left ventricular).

○ **sudden death**
    ○ diagnosis by autopsy but in some IHD can only be a presumptive diagnosis since there may be no naked eye evidence of myocardial infarction.

○ **acute myocardial infarction**
    ○ clinical, i.e. pulse, BP, lungs, shock
    ○ e.c.g.
    ○ cardiac enzymes, i.e. SCK, SGOT and SLDH (in first 2–3 days only).

○ **angina**
    ○ assess by history of response to degrees of effort
    ○ clinical examination
    ○ full blood check
    ○ blood cholesterol and triglycerides
    ○ urinalysis
    ○ e.c.g. at risk of little value
    ○ e.c.g. on exercise may be of value
    ○ therapeutic response to nitrates.

○ **dysrhythmias**
    ○ may require 24 hour recording.

○ **heart failure**
    ○ clinical examination
    ○ chest X-ray
    ○ e.c.g.

Planned care	○ **patient and family**
	    ○ most important to emphasize risk factors and that prevention and good outcome are largely in hands of the patient through self-help.
	
	○ **GP**
	    ○ presymptomatic prevention
	    ○ early diagnosis
	    ○ decisions on referral to hospital – immediate or later
	    ○ decisions on assessment – how far should GP go?
	    ○ decisions on general management and advice
	    ○ decisions on specific therapies
	    ○ decisions on rehabilitation and long term care.
	
	○ **hospital**
	    ○ for **acute myocardial infarctions** – in uncomplicated cases can be discharged home within a week
	    ○ for **angina** – assessment for medical or surgical treatments
	    ○ long term follow-up is not necessary by hospitals.
	
	○ **community services**
	    ○ health education and information programmes
	    ○ home nursing care support for some patients
	    ○ assistance in rehabilitation and social security.

Principles of management	○ **prevention**
	   – risk factors should be noted and corrected,
	   – particularly,
	    ○ no smoking
	    ○ low fat diet and weight control
	    ○ regular exercise
	    ○ control of high blood pressure and diabetes
	    ○ special attention to familial hypercholesterol and triglyceride groups.
	
	○ **rehabilitation**
	    ○ optimistic encouragement
	    ○ early ambulation
	    ○ graded progressive exercises
	    ○ early return to work.
	
	○ **long term care**
	   – patients with present or past IHD should be seen at least once a year either by GP or practice nurse.
	
	○ **aims of management**
	    ○ prevent onset or progression of IHD
	    ○ control/correct symptoms and effects of IHD
	    ○ teach patient self-help
	
	○ **Acute myocardial infarction,** see p. 139
	○ **Dysrhythmias,** see p. 189
	○ **Heart failure,** see p. 137

○ Angina
  - ○ make **clinical assessment** of severity by history, i.e. what brings on pain? How frequent? How much self-help such as stopping smoking? What response to medication?
  - ○ **general advice** on how to walk (speed), extra care in cold weather, avoidance of emotional stresses, avoidance of large meals.
  - ○ if **medication** considered necessary the following should be used, possibly step by step.

○ Nitrates
  - ○ glyceryl trinitrate sublingual or other routes
  - ○ long acting isosorbide dinitrate.

○ β-Blockers
  - ○ if symptoms are not controlled by general measures and nitrates then β-blockers should be tried
  - ○ take care if history of asthma or heart failure.

○ Calcium–channel blockers
  - ○ act through peripheral and coronary vasodilation
  - ○ either use to supplement β-blockers or even before these are tried.

○ Coronary artery surgery
  - ○ probably required in about 10% of persons with angina
  - ○ indicated if medical treatment does not control angina
  - ○ should be considered more readily in younger patients particularly with unstable angina, even in recent onset.
  - ○ **coronary artery bypass graft** using saphenous veins is the common procedure but **percutaneous transluminal coronary angioplasty** by inserting coronary catheters with balloons to dilate narrowed segments is being developed.

E2　　Respiratory

Asthma

What is it

Episodic and transient wheezing and breathlessness that may end in permanent airways obstruction.

Up to 25% of children have wheezing episodes before the age of 10 but only one in four of them will have symptoms persisting beyond that age.

Asthma developing in childhood or early adult life is usually type I immediate hypersensitivity mediated by IgE (extrinsic asthma) whereas asthma developing later in life is characterized by a type III delayed hypersensitivity reaction mediated by IgG (intrinsic asthma) following a type 1 reaction but with no external allergens identifiable.

Significance

○ incidence – 2 per 1000 (5 new patients per year)
○ prevalence – 15 per 1000 (50 patients per GP)
○ probably 5% of people have been subjected to attacks of asthma at some time
○ is a cause of sudden and unexpected death and when attacks occur causes appreciable disability and interference with normal activities. Produces much anxiety among patients and relatives.
○ in about 5–10% of cases permanent disability ensues after 10–20 years.
○ genetic factors involved in development with triggering of attacks by allergies, infection, exercise, irritants, mechanical factors (deep breaths), chemicals, psychological factors.
○ majority of deaths occur outside hospital and in many cases terminal episode not considered serious by GP.

Is diagnosis accurate?

Are there definable causes or triggers and, if so, can they be prevented?

What investigations

How good is patient's psychological adjustment to asthma and can he be relied on to properly use, and not abuse, therapy?

What programme of management for now and the future?

Diagnostic/investigative considerations	
History	FH or PH atopy. Seasonal or diurnal (early morning dippers) variation. Occupation. Chronic night cough/wheeze. Wheeze with URTIs. Any provocative factors – foods, pets, exercise, dusting, drugs
Examination	Neither pitch nor loudness of wheeze is indicative of severity of obstruction. Hyperinflation, poor expansion, use of accessory muscles suggest severe obstruction. Structural changes in chest may arise from long term obstruction
Lung function tests	Confirm degree of airways obstruction and confirm its reversibility. Allows objective monitoring of progress and PEFR should be regarded as a routine part of each clinical examination. FEV_1 and FVC may be used as assessment criteria if practice has vitelograph
Chest X-ray	Exclusion of other lung conditions – otherwise of little value
Eosinophils	In blood or sputum may be found in type I especially if associated aspergillosis
Prick skin testing	No value in diagnosis but may demonstrate allergenic cause to patient and improve compliance. Negative results may allow diagnosis of type III which has treatment/prognosis implications
Response to steroids	Refractory obstruction responds to several days of high dose steroids while irreversible obstruction will not

Planned care

Hospital management (urgent)
For severe acute attacks:

Clinical signs of danger
O sudden decrease exercise tolerance (decline in PEFR readings) O difficulty in speaking O use of accessory muscles O tachycardia > 110 (in absence of sympathomimetics) O pulsus paradoxus O PEFR < 100 litres/min O 'silent' chest (absence adventitious sounds due to overinflation)
<div align="center">ADMIT AS EMERGENCY</div>

GP management
O treat effectively and with confidence to minimize psychological problems.
O educate patient (and patients/family) to promote good understanding of nature of disease, course, prognosis, likely therapy and how to manage acute attacks. Emphasize which therapy preventive and which for symptomatic relief
O rationally plan drug therapy to use as few drugs as possible at any one time
O regularly monitor PEFR (teach patient to use peak flow meter at home)

Acute attack – see page 136

Chronic asthma

AVOID	Known allergens and trigger factors
Desensitization	On whole unsuccessful. May help if clearly provoked by pollens or moulds. No evidence mite desensitization of value
Disodium cromoglycate	Stabilizes mast cell membrane so stops type I reaction with release histamine etc.
	Works in $^2/_3$ children but much less in adults. Preventive only and will stop exercise induced attacks if taken before exercise starts.
	Trial for $^2/_{12}$ with plain (**not** Co variety) and keep record of number of attacks. If not effective then stop
Steroid aerosols	Provide maintenance steroid therapy (2 puffs q.i.d. $\equiv$ 7–10 mg prednisolone) without same likelihood of systemic side effects as oral therapy.
	Valueless for treatment of severe attack as action not immediate and cannot be inhaled deeply if bronchoconstriction present. For latter reason those on this therapy must have supply of oral prednisolone to switch to (at least 20 mg per day for 3 or 4 days) at onset of lower respiratory infection or increased breathlessness
Oral prednisolone	Used in severe cases. Start at 40–60 mg daily and after 3–5 days (when responding) cut by 5 mg every 3 days until minimum effective maintenance dose. If maintenance of about 5–10 mg per day then should be able to transfer to aerosol.
	If not then prednisolone on alternate days cuts risk of long term side effects.
	If no effect within 7 days of starting then therapy should be stopped as obstruction irreversible.
Oral antispasmodics	Work much better in early stages of acute attack than over long periods.

Alleviation of symptoms	Self-referral of patient should be encouraged early especially when bronchodilator aerosols are no longer effective.

Oral	Theophylline derivatives, e.g. Phyllocontin, Choledyl, Thean are effective but may cause nausea and vomiting
	Sympathomimetics, e.g. Ventolin, Alupent, Bricanyl act by stimulating β-adrenergic receptors in the bronchial wall and will often produce muscle tremors
	These groups are working at different intracellular sites and may have valuable additive effects
	In general longer to act, less effective, more side effects than aerosols
Aerosol bronchodilators	Sympathomimetics with rapid relief of symptoms MUST tell patient not to exceed the required dose which should be stated in terms of the number of inhalations at one time, the frequency of dosage and the maximum number of doses allowed in 24 hours. In acute exacerbation aerosol delivery is impaired and oral or parenteral therapy obligatory NB the dose of active drug varies in different aerosol preparations
Steroids	If on steroid aerosol therapy then MUST switch to oral therapy with onset of wheezing Remember that in acute attacks action of oral steroids is **slow** and i.v. steroids may be needed
Antibiotics	If attack is associated with infection then appropriate antibiotic should be given
Rectal Aminophylline	Often of value for the prevention of nocturnal symptoms. If used over prolonged period may give proctitis
Nebulizers	Will deliver high dosage of inhaled drugs. May lead to overdosage

Self-help
○ lead as normal a life as possible
○ avoid precipitating factors where possible
○ use drugs sensibly without abusing them
○ do **not** underestimate the severity of an attack and seek medical help early rather than late

Chronic Bronchitis

What is it

Epidemiologically defined as existing in any person who regularly expectorates sputum for at least 3 months of the year and has done so for 2 years. Once this is established there is an increased liability to acute chest infections and variable but progressive reduction of respiratory efficiency leading to severe respiratory failure in some. Pathologically the primary feature is the increased secretion of sticky mucus caused by hypertrophy of the mucous glands and an increase in size and number of the goblet cells.

Significance

Commonest chronic chest disorder seen in general practice with 20% of males and 5% of females over the age of 40 having symptoms to justify this diagnosis.

In any year in a practice of 2500
○ 100 will consult GP
○ 60 will be simple cases
○ 30 will suffer acute infective episodes
○ 10 will be invalids
○ 5 will be hospitalized
○ 2 will die

Risk factors
○ constitutional predisposition
○ increasing age
○ males (females increasing prevalence with smoking)
○ urban living/atmospheric pollution
○ social class IV and V
○ occupational dust and fumes
○ cigarette smoking

Important causes of morbidity and mortality
○ 50% persistent cough but no appreciable functional disability
○ 25% moderately disabled with recurrent chest infections, increasing absences from work and appreciable loss of respiratory function
○ 25% severely disabled over 5–10 year period

Early diagnosis possible in smokers with morning cough and decreased PEFR during exacerbation. Attention to risk factors at this stage may have some effect on future disability.

Special risk of developing progressive airways obstruction in
○ those with FH chronic bronchitis
○ heavy smokers who inhale deeply
○ those with a history of recurrent bronchitis during childhood or adulthood

Assessment

Is the diagnosis accurate?
○ late onset asthma
○ carcinoma lung
○ TB (in old men)
○ chronic left-sided heart failure
○ chronic chest disease, e.g. bronchiectasis, pneumoconioses

What is the functional state?
By the use of peak flow meter or Vitalograph the GP can identify those with irreversible airways obstruction that has not given rise to breathlessness. Disability is seldom found in patients with PEF>250 l/min.

Are there any risk factors present that may be alleviated?
○ stop smoking at any stage
○ occupational history
○ reduce overweight

Investigations
○ chest X-ray – initially to exclude other chronic chest disease and periodi- cally in heavy smokers to exclude carcinoma
○ PEFR/lung function – initially to assess degree of obstruction and regu- larly thereafter to provide objective assessment of disability
○ sputum culture – to exclude TB. Of limited value in exacerbations since findings do not often help in deciding choice of antibiotic (assume infection with predominantly *H.influenzae* or *Strep. pneumoniae*)

Planned care

Hospital management
○ during acute exacerbations may need admission for social or medical reasons. Especially in those developing any degree of respiratory failure (shallow respiration, cyanosis, drowsiness, headache, irritability, coarse tremor——▶admit as emergency)
○ referral to local chest physician may result in a more comprehensive degree of care than the GP can offer, if GP denied open access to physiotherapy department

GP management

○ forceful anti-smoking propaganda during or immediately after an acute exacerbation
○ demonstration of decreased function on peak flow meter
○ regular follow-up and review of chronic cases with disability

Antibiotics	Start course of treatment with appropriate antibiotic. Consider: 1. increasing resistance of *H.influenzae* to co-trimoxazole and the ampicillins, 2. penetration of antibiotic into sputum especially in chronic cases, 3. supply patients with antibiotics to take at first sign of flare-up (yellow sputum). No evidence that long term antibiotic therapy reduces number of exacerbations though may shorten duration.
Bronchodilators	Only helpful if element of reversible airways obstruction present can be continued by inhaler, orally or by suppository
Corticosteroids	Asthmatic type of bronchitis may respond well to oral steroids. Should only be given if objective evidence of benefit
Oxygen	Only for relief of hypoxia and only at low concentration (e.g. 24% by Venturi mask). Use for short periods has no demonstrable therapeutic benefit. Can be prescribed on FP 10
Physiotherapy	Usually only available at hospital. Can help in assisting patient clear his chest of sticky mucus
Diuretics	Needed for treatment of cor pulmonale which may develop

○ Consider problems of rehabilitation and employment (light job at work or disablement register or early retirement)
○ Consider need for rehousing and social services aid and assistance that may be given (home helps, meals on wheels, financial supplements, social visiting, etc.)

Self-help

○ stop smoking
○ do not go out in cold and damp weather
○ maintain an even temperature in the home.

Hay fever

What is it
Seasonal exposure to grass pollens or, more rarely, tree pollens or moulds producing a hypersensitivity reaction of the respiratory tract.

Significance
- at one time or another will affect 7% of the population especially those with a family history of atopy
- prevalence – 15 per 1000 (30–40 patients will be seen in a season)
- usually begins in teens or twenties with annual seasonal symptoms for some 5–15 years before natural resolution occurs.
- source of discomfort and personal misery but not a significant cause of morbidity and in no way life threatening

Assessment
- good clinical history (nasal obstruction, excess nasal discharge, sneezing, irritation of the eyes and sometimes wheezing) of symptoms between May and August gives diagnosis
- skin testing of little value

Planned care

Hospital management
- may need referral for removal associated nasal polyps

GP management
- social factors, e.g. type of employment, driving, important forthcoming events are as important as severity of symptoms in deciding therapy
- disadvantages of proposed treatment must be fully explained to patient

Antihistamines	Trial of different compounds may be necessary to find most suitable one for patient. Side effects may be appreciable. **Must warn re driving, using machinery**
Disodium cromoglycate	Regular nasal inhalation may help some patients though treatment is expensive and tedious
Local steroids	Costly and not always well tolerated though this can be very successful in some patients
Systemic steroids	Use of such powerful drugs for a benign condition is only justified for severe symptoms (including asthma) or to tide patient over an important event. Can be orally for a short time or single injection of depot preparation. NB full explanation/**Steroid card**
Desensitization	Preseasonal courses over 2–3 years will give complete control in about $1/3$ of cases. Expensive and time consuming with serious risk of sudden collapse, shock and even death

Self-help

○ accept that all symptoms don't need drug therapy and that treatment may well be more dangerous than original condition

○ avoid high pollen concentration where possible (long grass; car or train journeys with open windows; house windows open on hot, humid, windy days)

○ do not go camping

○ do not walk through long grass

E3 Rheumatic

Ankylosing Spondylitis

What is it

A **chronic arthritis** which:
○ mainly affects the spine and sacro-iliac joints
○ usually runs a prolonged course
○ causes chronic backache and permanent stiffening of the spine

Characterized by
○ inflammation of the spinal joints (lower thoracic and lumbar)
○ sacroilitis
○ ligamentous calcification
○ high prevalence of HLA-B27 histocompatibility antigen

Cause
○ not known   – possible auto-immunity

Significance

○ incidence   – 1 per 10 000 (1 new patient per GP every 5 years)
○ prevalence   – 1 per 2000 (1 per GP)
○ sex distribution – Males>>Females
○ age of onset   – usually under 30 years, may occur up to 50 years
○ course   – usually good with treatment
                  – small proportion (<10%) develop serious systemic complications

Methods of prevention

Nil known
  – ? genetic counselling

Opportunities for early diagnosis

Clinical acumen
e.g. beware of labelling young man with persistent stiff back as a malingerer or a neurotic – he may have ankylosing spondylitis

Diagnostic features

Onset
○ usually insidious
○ occasionally acute

Back pain
○ diffuse or localized to lumbosacral area
○ worse in morning
○ may develop pain in thoracic or cervical spine later
○ may radiate to buttocks

Stiffness
○ worse in morning
○ improves with exercise
○ limited mobility on examination

Associated arthritis
○ involvement of small joints uncommon
○ may affect hips or knees

Systemic disturbances (usually absent)
○ malaise
○ fatigue
○ loss of weight
○ fever

Other manifestations
○ depression
○ enteropathic colitis ⎫
○ Reiter's syndrome ⎬ may represent
○ psoriasis   ⎭ separate entities
○ iritis
○ vavular heart disease
○ respiratory failure

Investigations
○ ESR usually raised (may be normal)
○ R.A. latex, Rose–Waaler or similar
　　　○ persistently negative
○ full blood count normal
○ HLA-B27 antigen present in over 90% of cases
○ radiology
　　　○ may be negative initially
　　　○ sacroilitis
　　　○ progressive calcification of ligaments ⟶ bamboo spine

Planned care

Patient
○ understanding of condition
○ compliance with therapy
○ exercise, especially swimming

GP
○ confirm diagnosis
○ assess patient
○ choose therapy
○ consider referral
○ review regularly

Hospital
○ confirmation of diagnosis
○ support and reassurance
○ advice on long term arrangement

Community Services
○ employment
　　　○ DRO
　　　○ house alterations

Principles of management

Relief of pain and suppression of inflammation
○ drug therapy
　　　○ analgesics
　　　○ NSAIDs
　　　○ steroids may be dramatically beneficial if condition uncontrolled.
　　　　　Use minimum dosage for as short a time as possible
○ radiotherapy no longer recommended – because of risks of leukaemia
　　later
○ avoid bed rest

Relief of stiffness, improvement of mobility and prevention of spinal deformity
○ own exercises – regular and intensive
○ physiotherapy
○ breathing exercises
○ surgery rarely required

Gout

What is it

An **acute arthritis** which:
○ usually affects only one or two joints
○ has an acute onset
○ causes severe localized pain

Chronic gout may lead to renal damage and arthritis
Characterized by
○ crystal deposition (uric acid)
○ foreign-body inflammatory reaction of synovium, synovial fluids and articular cartilage

Caused by
○ hyperuricaemia
    ○ primary (↓excretion of uric acid)
    ○ secondary to
        ○ leukaemias
        ○ chronic renal failure
        ○ drugs, e.g. diuretics
        ○ hyperparathyroidism

Significance

○ incidence   –   0.5 per 1000 (1 new patient per GP per year)
○ prevalence   –   2 per 1000 (5 patients per GP)
○ sex distribution   –   males>>females (10:1)
○ age of onset   –   40 years onwards
○ course   –   eminently treatable

Methods of prevention

○ prophylactic use of allopurinol in conditions predisposing to gout
○ care in prescribing certain drugs i.e. diuretics

Opportunities for early diagnosis

○ clinical acumen, e.g. consider all sudden painful joints in middle-aged men as gout

Diagnostic features

Onset
○ sudden in acute cases

Arthritis
○ single joint
○ most often big toe
○ reddening of skin over affected joint

Tophi
○ over joints
○ on the ears
○ in the nasal cartilage
○ late and not common

Underlying disease
○ e.g. treated leukaemia

Underlying drugs
○ e.g. thiazides

Renal colic
○ uric acid calculi (uncommon)

Renal failure and hypertension
○ due to nephropathy (rare)

Investigations

- O serum uric acid >0.4 mmol (on at least two occasions). Can be normal during attack
- O full blood count
    - O may be slight leukocytosis
- O urine
    - O for albumin and blood
- O blood urea and creatinine
    - O normal, unless renal failure
- O serum calcium, phosphate and alkaline phosphatase
    - O to exclude hyperparathyroidism
- O radiology (often negative in early case)
    - O tophaceous osteolysis
    - O topaceous bone formation
    - O soft tissue swelling with periarticular calcification
    - O calcareous deposits in kidneys
- O synovial fluid
    - O monosodium urate crystals demonstrated by polarized light microscopy

Planned care

Patient
- O understanding of condition and trigger factors
- O compliance with therapy

GP
- O confirm diagnosis
- O choose therapy
- O consider referral
- O review regularly

Hospital
- O management of refractory and complicated cases

Community Services
- O district nurse
- O dietician

Principles of management

Relief of pain and suppression of inflammation
- O rest
- O cradle
- O drugs
    - O NSAIDS
    - O ACTH 40 units 6 hourly initially
    - O colchicine now rarely used.

Reduction of serum uric acid (maintain below 0.3 mmol)
- O allopurinol 300 – 600 mg daily
- O probenecid (not in renal failure)
- O add small dose of anti-inflammatory drug for first 4 weeks to prevent acute attacks

General advice
- O low purine diets are unnecessary
- O avoid crash diets in the obese
- O avoid excessive alcohol
- O avoid infections, operations, trauma and certain drugs

Osteoarthritis (Osteoarthrosis)

What is it

A **degenerative joint disease of uncertain cause**
Predisposed by
○ chronic trauma
○ obesity
○ occupational

Characterized by
○ hydroxyapatite crystals in cartilage leading to inflammatory reaction
○ osteophyte formation
○ joint deformity and displacement

Significance

○ disease of ageing — 95% of people over 65 have OA somewhere (radiologically)
○ prevalence — 25 per 1000 (62 patients per GP)
 — many cases not reported to doctor (patient accepts symptoms)
○ sex distribution — 2 females : 1 male
○ course — usually slow progression but not necessarily so

Methods of prevention

○ weight control
○ prevention of trauma to joints
○ effective treatment of joint injury and underlying joint diseases

Opportunities for early diagnosis

○ clinical acumen and awareness
 NOTE
 referred pains from affected joints
 e.g. hip———▶knee, spine———▶leg

Diagnostic features

Painful impairment of function
○ usually affects one joint predominantly
○ pain usually on movement
○ pain in response to weight-bearing
○ pain at maximum range of movement
○ movement of joint restricted
○ worse at end of day

Crepitus
○ palpable (in superficial joints)

Pattern of arthritis
○ hands (especially distal IP joints)
○ feet
○ knees
○ shoulders   Descending
○ cervical spine   order
○ elbows   of
○ lumbar spine   frequency
○ wrists   affected

Joint and muscle stiffness
○ particularly after rest ('joints get set')

Diagnostic features continued	**Swelling and deformity**
	 ○ effusion
	 ○ synovial thickening
	 ○ osteophyte formation
	 ○ Heberden's nodes
	
	 Investigations
	 ○ full blood count and ESR (=normal)
	 ○ radiology
	     ○ marginal osteophytes
	     ○ narrowing of the joint space
	     ○ densification of subchondral bone
	     ○ remodelling of joint (late)
	 ○ synovial fluid
	     ○ clear, amber, normal viscosity
	     ○ few leukocytes
	     ○ normal enzymes

Planned care	**Patient**
	 ○ understanding condition
	 ○ rest and exercise as advised
	 ○ weight reduction where necessary
	
	 GP
	 ○ confirm diagnosis
	 ○ reassure patient that unlikely to be progressive and crippling
	 ○ choose therapy
	 ○ consider referral
	
	 Hospital
	 ○ specialist opinion ? surgery
	 ○ physiotherapy
	 ○ occupational therapy
	 ○ rheumatologist's support for patient
	
	 Community Services
	 ○ district nurse, health visitor
	 ○ social services
	     ○ aids
	     ○ day care
	     ○ residential care
	     ○ casework
	 ○ employment services
	     ○ DRO
	 ○ financial support
	     ○ Social Security
	     ○ disabled housewife's allowance
	     ○ mobility allowance
	     ○ attendance allowance

Principles of
management

General measures to prevent deterioration
○ weight reduction
○ avoidance of trauma
    ○ work
    ○ sport
○ use of stick and other aids

Pain relief
○ drug therapy – analgesics and NSAIDs
○ local steroid injections
○ physiotherapy
○ surgery
    ○ osteotomy
    ○ arthrodesis
    ○ joint replacement

Rehabilitation
○ physical
    ○ physiotherapy
○ psychosocial
    ○ occupational therapy
    ○ social therapy
    ○ employment

Polymyalgia Rheumatica

What is it

A **chronic myalgia** which:
○ mainly affects shoulder and hip girdles
○ runs a prolonged course
○ may be associated with cranial arteritis
○ may be secondary to malignant disease
○ in old persons

Characterized by
○ ? inflammatory changes in affected muscles
○ arteritis, especially temporal which may lead to blindness (often sub-clinical)

Caused by
○ ? autoimmune disorder

Significance

○ incidence   – 1 per 3–4000 (1 new patient per GP every 1–2 years)
○ prevalence   – 1 per 2–3000 (1 patient per GP)
○ age of onset – over 60
○ course   – long duration, year or longer
                  – good response to treatment with steroids
                  – risk of **sudden blindness** if associated cranial arteritis not adequately controlled

Methods of prevention

Nil known

Opportunities for early diagnosis

Clinical acumen, e.g. generalized stiffness and pains in neck and back, worse on rising in morning

Diagnostic features

Onset
○ usually acute
○ occasionally insidious

Pain and stiffness
○ shoulder and hip girdles and back and neck affected
○ prolonged morning stiffness

Associated symptoms
○ malaise and depression
○ headache
○ visual problems – beware temporal arteritis

Exclude possible underlying neoplasia, e.g. cancers of breast, lung, or prostate, myeloma

Investigations
○ ESR>50mm/h (if very high consider arteritis or myelomatosis)
○ FBC – often low haemoglobin
○ serum proteins – raised globulin (exclude myelomatosis)
○ chest X-ray (to exclude underlying disease)
○ R.A. latex or similar (to exclude seropositive arthritis)
○ biopsy temporal artery if indicated

Planned care	**Patient and family** ○ understanding of condition ○ compliance with therapy **GP** ○ confirm diagnosis ○ advise patient ○ choose therapy ○ consider referral – most uncomplicated cases can be managed by GP ○ review regularly **Hospital** ○ specialist opinion – if possible arteritis **Community Services** ○ home help ○ aids } during acute phase ○ district nurse
Principles of management	**Relief of pain and stiffness** ○ steroids (20 mg or more prednisolone daily initially – reduce gradually but continue for year or longer) ○ analgesics **Prevent serious complication, i.e. temporal arteritis** ○ close observation (if suspected) ○ **immediate** high-dose steroids (50 mg prednisone daily) ○ **then** urgent referral for biopsy and advice

Suggested drug treatment in the management of polymyalgia rheumatica

Drug	Dose	Route of administration
Prednisolone	Large doses of up to 60 mg or more daily at first and once controlled go onto a maintenance dose of 5–10 mg daily. Steroids should be continued for a year or longer	Oral

Rheumatoid Arthritis

What is it

A **chronic polyarthritis** which:
○ mainly affects the peripheral joints
○ usually runs a prolonged course
○ exhibits exacerbations and remissions
○ may be accompanied by general systemic disturbances

Characterized by
○ inflammation/swelling of synovial membrane and periarticular tissue
○ subchondral osteoporosis
○ erosion of cartilage and bone
○ wasting of associated muscles
○ pain is worse in morning

Caused by
○ ? autoimmune disorder

Significance

○ incidence   —   1 per 1000 (2–3 new patients per GP per year)
○ prevalence   —   5–8 per 1000 (12–20 patients per GP)
○ sex distribution —   3 females : 1 male
○ age of onset   —   childhood———→old age. Usually 25–55 years
○ course   —   long duration, usually years
                   —   30% become severely disabled
                   —   30% become moderately disabled
                   —   30% become mildly disabled
                   —   10% have no disability
                   —   a few patients die of the disease

**Methods of
prevention**

Nil known

**Opportunities for
early diagnosis
Diagnostic
features**

Clinical acumen – often commences in a single joint with general malaise

Precusors
○ carpal tunnel syndrome
○ fleeting joint pains
○ transient muscle stiffness
○ generally 'off colour' and depression

Onset
○ normally insidious
○ occasionally acute

Pattern of arthritis
○ often symmetrical
○ proximal M–P joints
○ wrists   descending
○ knees   order
○ elbows   of
○ shoulders   frequency
○ foot joints   affected
○ hips
○ neck

Diagnostic features continued	**joint and muscle stiffness**
	○ characteristically prolonged after sleep or inactivity
	    i.e. worse in mornings
	
	limitation of movement
	swelling and deformity
	○ ulnar deviation
	○ spindling of fingers
	
	systemic disturbances (20% of cases)
	○ anorexia
	○ weight loss
	○ fatigue
	○ malaise
	○ sweating
	○ tachycardia
	
	subcutaneous nodules (10–20% of cases)
	other manifestations, e.g. uveitis, vasculitis, neuropathy, lymphadenopathy, amyloid
	Investigations:
	○ ESR raised in active stages
	○ R.A. Latex, Rose–Waaler or similar
	    ○ positive in 80% eventually
	    ○ high titres⟶bad prognosis
	○ full blood count
	    ○ hypochromic
	    ○ normocytic anaemia
	    ○ mild polymorphonuclear leukocytosis
	○ plasma protein pattern
	    ○ increased globulin
	    ○ decreased albumin
	○ radiology
	    ○ demineralization of bone-ends (early)
	    ○ narrowing of joint space
	    ○ marginal erosions
	    ○ secondary osteoarthritis (late)
	○ synovial fluid
	    ○ turbid, yellow/green, diminished viscosity
	    ○ many leukocytes
	    ○ raised enzymes

Planned care	**Patient and family** ○ understanding of condition ○ knowledge of services available (Arthritis & Rheumatism Council Handbook, 41 Eagle Street, London WC1R 4AR) ○ rest and exercise as advised ○ compliance with therapy **GP** ○ confirm diagnosis ○ assess patient and family ○ choose therapy ○ consider referral ○ review regularly ○ optimistic support

Planned care
continued

Hospital
○ admission
○ specialist opinion
○ physiotherapy
○ occupational therapy
○ social work support

Community Services
○ district nurse
○ health visitor
○ social services
    ○ structural alterations to house
    ○ day care
    ○ aids
    ○ residential care
    ○ casework

Employment Services
○ DRO

Financial support
○ social security
○ attendance allowance
○ disabled housewife's allowance
○ mobility allowance

Principles of management

Relief of pain and suppression of inflammation
○ bed rest
○ splints
○ drug therapy
○ local steroid injections
○ synovectomy

Maintenance of general health
○ diet
○ specific therapy

Maintenance of function and correction of deformity
○ splints
○ physiotherapy
○ occupational therapy
○ surgery

Rehabilitation
○ physical
○ psychological
○ physiotherapy
○ occupational therapy
○ social therapy
○ employment

Specific drug therapy

First line
Objective to relieve pain and stiffness with analgesic and anti-inflammatory drugs.
○ aspirin and salicylates
○ other non-steroid anti-inflammatory drugs.

Second line
Specific in affecting the rheumatoid process. Slow effects – may take 4–6 months for full benefits. Risks of side effects greater than with first line drugs.
○ gold
○ penicillamine
○ chloroquine – retinopathy unlikely if recommended doses not exceeded

Third line
Corticosteroids have immunosuppressant and anti-inflammatory actions.
○ **Systemically** may produce dramatic quick benefits but, if used long term, side effects and complications are almost inevitable.
○ **Intra-articular injections** may relieve pain, reduce swelling and increase mobility.

Fourth line
Immunosuppressants if no response to other therapy
○ azathioprine
○ chlorambucil
○ methotrexate.
They must only be used under strict controls with blood checks every 2–3 weeks.

E4 CNS

Epilepsy

What is it

Epilepsy is a symptom and not a disease.
It is characterized by recurrent paroxysmal disorders of brain function which produce a fit or seizure, either focal or generalized, usually accompanied by a disturbance of consciousness.

Type	Characteristics
Grand mal	By far the commonest type. Sudden loss of consciousness with tonic phase followed by clonic phase and postical drowsiness or confusion
Petit mal	Condition of childhood with tendency to remit in adolescence. Always idiopathic. Frequent brief interruptions of consciousness with immediate recovery and no sequelae

Focal epilepsy
  Motor
 	
  Sensory
  Temporal lobe
	Nature of attack depends on primary site of lesion
	Jacksonian seizure. May be short lived weakness of part involved in fit (Tod's paralysis)
	As motor but originating in precentral cortex
	Complex disorders of sensation which may be followed by generalized fits

Febrile fits	Affects 3% of children Defined as fit associated with axillary temperature of over 38°C 1 in 5 will go on to have afebrile attacks

Significance

○ incidence – less than 1 per 1000 (1 new patient every 2–3 years)
○ prevalence – 3 per 1000 of the population (7–10 patients per GP)
○ in 95% of cases is idiopathic
○ diagnosis carries far reaching social consequences and should not be made unless there is definite evidence for it.
○ generally life long condition which requires long term anticonvulsant therapy and also management and care of many social problems of suitable employment and acceptance by general population
○ however, a proportion (about one quarter) will cease to suffer attacks

Assessment

Ideally all presenting cases should be referred for hospital assessment (e.e.g. etc) to exclude any potentially remediable organic neurological disease and to confirm the diagnosis.

Planned care

Hospital management
O for initial investigation and confirmation of diagnosis
O referral if control difficulties or serious mental or physical difficulties

GP management
O information
O reassurance
O instruction
O regular review

Anticonvulsant therapy
O anticonvulsant drugs are semispecific in their effects on different types of epilepsy
O one drug should be used alone whenever possible with its dose being adjusted to yield a serum concentration within the accepted therapeutic range. Aim is to achieve optimum control with minimum of adverse effects.
O important to avoid polytherapy as interactions with antiepileptic drugs occur frequently
O patient understanding of condition and aims of therapy is essential as poor compliance is a major control problem

Self-help
O comprehension and insight into condition essential
O avoidance of potentially dangerous situations (working at heights, or with machinery, swimming alone, driving within 3 years of last fit, etc.) while leading as normal a life as possible
O information from
British Epilepsy Association,
3–6 Alfred Place,
London WC1E 7ED
O local groups for support and mutual aid

Planned care
continued

Type of epilepsy	Drugs of choice	Dosage	Adverse effects
Grand mal	Phenytoin (first choice especially in the young and old)	Start 200 mg once daily in adults or up to 8 mg/kg in children. Serum levels in 2–4 weeks with adjustment of dosage to produce level in optimum range 40–80 μmol/l	Rashes gingival hyperplasia coarse facies acne hirsutism megaloblastic anaemia rarely hypocalcaemia and osteomalacia
	Phenobarbitone (poorly tolerated by children)	Limit dose to 120 mg per day in adults. Half-life of 2–6 days so give as one dose at night. Therapeutic serum range 42–105 μmol/l	Rashes Depression of cognitive functions and memory, rarely megaloblastic anaemia
especially if with difficult personality traits	Carbamazepine (may be tried in chronic epilepsy if other drugs have failed)	200 mg once or twice daily in adults (100 mg children) increasing to maximum of 20 mg/kg. Therapeutic serum range 15–50 μmol/l	diplopia nystagmus drowsiness/dizziness ataxia nausea/vomiting aplastic anaemia
	Sodium valproate	Will control but probably not as effective as standard drugs	
Petit mal	Ethosuximide (drug of choice)	Start 250 mg once daily increasing as necessary to a maximum of 30 mg/kg	Drowsiness Gastric upset
	Sodium valproate (is active against grand mal seizures which may co-exist)	Start 200 mg b.d. regardless of age (as long as over 3 years old)	Nausea Transient hair loss Occasional tremor Thrombocytopenia
Temporal lobe (other partial seizures treated with same range of drugs as primary grand mal)	Sulthiame	Start 100 mg b.d. in adults 3–5 mg/kg in divided doses in children. 200 mg t.i.d. optimum in adults	Drowsiness Paraesthesia Overbreathing
	Carbamazepine	More useful in temporal lobe than Grand mal	
Myoclonic seizures	A variety of syndromes in childhood occur with myoclonic jerking. **Sodium valproate** (first choice) and **Clonazepam** are effective		

Migraine

What is it

Symptom complex of uncertain cause

Headache
○ unilateral or bilateral
○ intermittent and recurrent

Visual
○ may be preceded or associated with visual disturbances

GI symptoms
○ often anorexia, nausea, vomiting

Significance

○ incidence — 3 per 1000 (7–8 new patients per year)
○ prevalence — 20 per 1000 (50 patients per GP)
○ age of onset — usually starts in childhood, adolescence or early adult life
○ course — tendency for attacks to go on for 10–15 years and then become less frequent

Assessment

○ diagnosis
    — on clinical grounds (see chart)
    — any persistent neurological signs demand further investigation
    — local examination to exclude pain from:
        ○ cervical spine
        ○ paranasal sinuses
        ○ eyes
        ○ hypertension

○ trigger factors (see chart)
○ other causes of similar headaches
    tension headaches
    intracranial lesions, e.g. aneurysm, tumours

Planned care

Patient and self-care
Knowledge of possible '**trigger factors**' and subsequent avoidance

○ anxiety	○ fatigue	○ travel
○ worry	○ stooping	○ climate
○ emotion	○ lifting	○ sunshine
○ depression	○ late rising	○ glare
○ shock	○ hypoglycaemia	○ visual strain
○ excitement	○ alcohol	○ noise
○ change of routine	○ hypnotics	○ smells
○ foods	○ pre- and para-	
— chocolate	menstrum	
— citrus fruit	○ hypertension	
— cheese		
— pastry		
— fried food		

Understanding of **personal prodromata** and institution of prompt self-treatment

Visual
- ○ diplopia
- ○ failure to focus
- ○ scotomata
- ○ scintillata (lights, spots, lines, colours)

Neurological
- ○ vertigo
- ○ paraesthesiae
- ○ paralysis
- ○ yawning
- ○ trembling
- ○ weakness
- ○ dysarthria
- ○ pallor
- ○ hemiplegia
- ○ ophthalmoplegia

Psychological
- ○ depression
- ○ irritability
- ○ anxiety
- ○ excessive well-being
- ○ excitability
- ○ talkativeness

Physiological
- ○ weight gain
- ○ oedema
- ○ diuresis

Patient should:
- ○ keep diary
- ○ understand pattern of attacks
- ○ prevent where possible
- ○ self treat early

GP + disease management
- ○ help patient to understand and manage his/her own problem
- ○ confirm diagnosis
- ○ exclude serious disease
- ○ prescribe, if necessary (see list)

Preventive drugs	Clonidine Propranolol Methysergide Pizotifen
Analgesics	Aspirin Paracetamol
Tranquillizing muscle relaxants	Diazepam
Specific drugs	Ergotamine
Antiemetics	Metoclopramide Prochlorperazine

Hospital and other sources

○ **referral** if persistent neurological signs
○ **referral** if frequent, severe, debilitating attacks uncontrolled by usual measures
○ **referral** for social, emotional or financial help, if indicated.
○ Migraine Trust and British Migraine Association provide:
    ○ help and advice to sufferers
    ○ promote research
    ○ promote education

○ The Migraine Trust, 42 Great Ormonde Street, London WC1N 3HD.
○ British Migraine Association, 178A High Street, Weybridge, Surrey KT14 7ED.

Clinical types

Clinical types	Prodromata	Headache	Associated symptoms	Signs	Notes
Common migraine	nil	Often unilateral	Anorexia, nausea, vomiting	nil	♀ > ♂
Classical migraine	visual, paraesthesiae, ophthalmoplegia, hemiplegia, dysarthria, tinnitus, ataxia	Usually unilateral	Anorexia, nausea, vomiting	nil	♀ > ♂
Symptomatic migraine	Any of above	Strictly unilateral	Anorexia, nausea, vomiting	Persistent Neurological	Beware late onset
Cluster headaches	nil	Unilateral Facial neuralgia	Unilateral – epiphora – nasal blockage	Unilateral red eye	♂ > ♀
Abdominal migraine	nil	Absent or mild	Abdominal pain anorexia, nausea vomiting ➔ketosis	nil	Usually children 'Periodic syndrome'
Tension headache	nil	Usually bilateral – top of head – frontal – occipital	nil	Localized Muscular	NOT responsive to ergotamine

Multiple Sclerosis

What is it

Relapsing and remitting disorder in which plaques of demyelination may affect any part of the white matter of the CNS

Symptoms due to demyelination are irreversible but as oedema in the surrounding tissue is reabsorbed there is a substantial return of function which may obscure the underlying deficit

Significance

○ peak age of onset 30 years
○ prevalence 1 per 1000 (2–3 patients per GP)
○ may be due to inherited predisposition causing CNS to react abnormally to a virus infection
○ very variable clinical course but onset at time of marriage/young family and average duration of about 25 years emphasizes the tremendous social as well as medical implications
○ early diagnosis may be difficult and no means of prevention or effective long term treatment

Assessment

Diagnosis is almost entirely a clinical problem

Presenting symptoms	Notes
Weakness (40% of cases)	Tiredness or heaviness of one or both legs due to spastic weakness. Accompanying dull ache and tendency to trip on rough ground. Upper motor neuron lesion on examination
Visual symptoms (40% of cases)	Optic neuritis. Loss of vision usually uniocular with ↓VA and central scotoma on examination. May see optic atrophy after about 1 month
Sensory symptoms (20% of cases)	Paraesthesia, dysaesthesia. Proprioceptive disorders with sensory ataxia and incoordination. Mild symptoms not always accompanied by signs
Brain stem syndromes	Vertigo, diplopia, facial palsy, dysarthria. Ataxic nystagmus highly suggestive of DS
Others	Rarely sphincter disturbances, dementia or euphoria/depression may occur early

No relevant GP investigations and all presenting cases should be seen by neurologist for confirmation of diagnosis.
Difficult to predict the clinical course in an individual patient.
○ benign – one or two attacks in lifetime
○ relapsing – increasingly poor recovery from successive relapses with significant disability within 10 years of onset
○ progressive – rapid progressive course
　　　　　　　 – premature death

Planned care	**Hospital management**
	O initial investigation/diagnosis
	O referral if unmanageable acute episode or serious mental or physical difficulties
	O in general, long term hospital care facilities for the young disabled are poor and community care has potentially far more to offer.

Hospital management
O initial investigation/diagnosis
O referral if unmanageable acute episode or serious mental or physical difficulties
O in general, long term hospital care facilities for the young disabled are poor and community care has potentially far more to offer.

GP management
After initial episode diagnosis may not be certain or, if it is, there may be prolonged remission so probably unwise to inform patient that he has MS. Once repeated episode, however, relatives and patient should be fully informed with (optimistic) explanation of implications.

During relapses

Rest	Sensible during attack but no real evidence avoiding undue fatigue will help stop relapse occurring
Antispasticity agents	Such as baclofen, dantrolene may help prevent painful spasms in bedbound patients
Physiotherapy	May improve ability to walk but of little value in acute or advanced disease
ACTH i.m. or prednisolone oral	No strong reason to prefer ACTH to prednisolone. Prednisolone 30 mg daily (descending over 2 weeks) hastens recovery from individual relapse but does not affect eventual outcome. Long term steroid therapy is of **no** value
Watch urinary tract	UTI very likely and important to keep urine sterile with antibiotics if appropriate. If recurrent infection then regular rotating antibiotic therapy may help. Urine incontinence may be helped by frequent visits to toilet and pressing abdominal wall to help emptying. Indwelling catheter may become necessary

Long term
O family needs help as well as patient
O primary care team involvement in trying to improve quality of life of patient and prevent loneliness and deprivation
e.g.
    O day centres
    O social gatherings for the handicapped
    O occupational therapy or sheltered employment
    O physical aids
    O home adaptions

Patient self-help
O determination to lead as normal a life as possible
O information and point of contact supplied by
    The Multiple Sclerosis Society,
    4 Tachbrook Street,
    London SW1V 1SJ
O local groups for support and aid.

Parkinsonism

What is it

An extrapyramidal disorder manifested by:
- tremor
- slowness of movement
- rigidity
- incidence 0.1 per 1000 (1 new case every 5 years per GP)
- prevalence 1–2 per 1000 (3–4 cases per GP)

- **clinical types**
    - idiopathic – cause of destruction of brain stem nuclei unknown
    - atherosclerotic – occurs in elderly with evidence of other major atherosclerotic disorders
    - drug induced – in psychiatric patients on long term phenothiazines particularly by injection and also in elderly patients treated for a variety of symptoms with phenothiazines
    - postencephalitic – very rare.

- **natural history**
    - condition of ageing, most cases arise after 60 years
    - progressive deterioration
    - drug induced – disappears when drugs stopped.

Significance

- probably 1 in 10 of over-65s suffers from some degree of parkinsonism.
- relentlessly progressive in spite of therapy.
- severe disabilities render victim almost helpless and in need of constant care at home or in an institution.
- long lasting, over 10 years with strains on carers.

Assessment

Clinical diagnosis and assessment.
- **early**
    - tremor
    - difficulty in writing
    - falls+
    - facial masking
    - loss of arm swing on walking
    - considerable independence
- **late**
    - increasing functional physical and mental disabilities
    - rigidity+
    - tremor+
    - shuffling stooping gait.

Planned care

- **early diagnosis** important, not because of success of treatment but in order to prepare patient and family for long term care.
- **family** must be informed of progressive nature of disorder, but with as much optimism as possible.
- **GP**
    - can commence drug therapy and advice on home conditions and aids.
    - regular surveillance and support.

○ **The Team**
  ○ home nurse will play an increasingly important role in the later stages
  ○ home nurse and social worker should get to know patient and family in early stages.

○ **Specialist**
  ○ to confirm diagnosis when necessary
  ○ to advise on therapy
  ○ to provide rehabilitative care
  ○ to admit to hospital or other unit when necessary.

Principles of management

○ inform patient and family with kindness and hope of nature of disorder and the therapies available
○ encourage self-help and independence
○ **step-by-step therapy** with drugs to improve quality of life and delay progression. Choice of —
  ○ **anticholinergics** to be tried first. Particularly useful in drug-induced parkinsonism.
  ○ **levodopa** first choice for disabled patients. Replenishes dopamine. More effective in younger (under 75) and recent-onset cases. Side effects may cause problems. Start with low doses and work up slowly. Do not stop abruptly. Slow improvement (over months) which may last for some years.
  ○ **amantadine** — may help a few patients in early stages. Few side effects.
  ○ **bromocriptine** — use only in those who cannot tolerate levodopa.
  ○ **surgery** — stereotactic thalmotomy said to relieve tremor and rigidity. Consider in those not responding to drug therapy. Relatively minor procedure in expert hands.

Self-help from
Parkinson's Disease Society,
36 Portland Place,
London W1N 3DG.

Stroke

What is it

Disturbance of the CNS resulting from an area of brain damage caused by decreased cerebral blood flow. Neurological dysfunction is generally of rapid onset and lasts for more than 1 hour.

Type	Pathophysiology	Presentation
Thrombo-embolic infarction	Accounts for over 50% of strokes. Arises from occlusion of arteries often already atheromateous. Extracranial vessel occlusion (especially in normotensives) and emboli from diseased carotids or heart are as important as primary intracranial occlusion	Often evolves over a period of hours and patient usually aware of progressive deficit. May have been preceded by brief focal neurological disturbances with abrupt onset and full recovery (transient ischaemic attacks)
Haemorr-hage	Especially in hypertensives. Vessel rupture and massive bleed or small microaneurysmic bleeds giving areas of brain softening. Rarely from blood diseases, SBE, anticoagulants	May be precipitated by exertion or emotion. Rapid onset with loss of consciousness in 50%. Hemiplegia or hemiparesis. Far higher mortality than infarction
	Subarachnoid haemorrhage	Sudden onset severe headache often rapidly into coma or fitting. Associated vomiting, neck stiffness and backache

Differential diagnosis: cerebral tumour (3–5% of those diagnosed as stroke); chronic subdural haematoma; hypertensive encephalopathy; cerebral abscess; meningococcal infection; hypoglycaemia.

Significance

○ incidence – annually 2–3 new cases per 1000 of the population (5–8 new patients per GP each year)
○ prevalence – 5–6 per 1000 (15–20 patients per GP)
○ 70% occur over the age of 70 but equal sex incidence
○ 50% die in the first month, 25% have severe disability and only 25% will recover with minor or no disability.
○ in GB about 100 000 are living with the residual effects of strokes imposing a tremendous social and management burden on their families and on the community
○ no effective treatment
○ prevention must be the GP's aim
○ early diagnosis and effective treatment of hypertension is the most hopeful measure that can be taken

Significance
continued

Risk factors in strokes

○ hypertension
○ cardiac disease
    ○ failure
    ○ ischaemic heart disease
    ○ embolic source   mural thrombosis
                             valvular vegetations
○ TIAs
○ previous strokes
○ increased haematocrit
○ lipid abnormalities (under age 55)
○ diabetes mellitus
○ smoking
○ oral contraceptive pill
○ family history

Assessment and
planned care

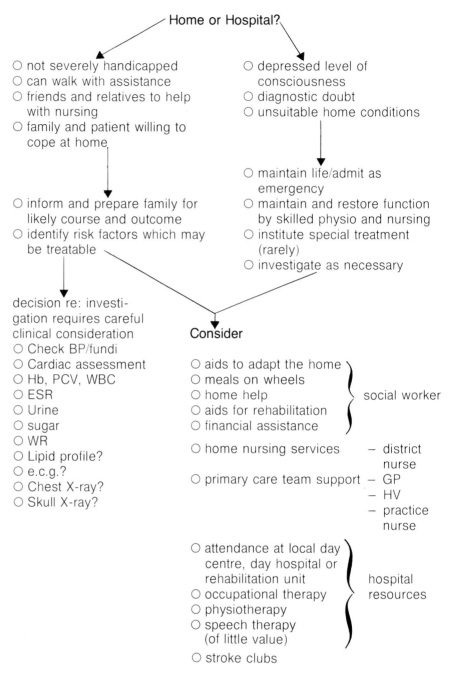

Home or Hospital?

○ not severely handicapped
○ can walk with assistance
○ friends and relatives to help
   with nursing
○ family and patient willing to
   cope at home

○ depressed level of
   consciousness
○ diagnostic doubt
○ unsuitable home conditions

○ inform and prepare family for
   likely course and outcome
○ identify risk factors which may
   be treatable

○ maintain life/admit as
   emergency
○ maintain and restore function
   by skilled physio and nursing
○ institute special treatment
   (rarely)
○ investigate as necessary

decision re: investi-
gation requires careful
clinical consideration
○ Check BP/fundi
○ Cardiac assessment
○ Hb, PCV, WBC
○ ESR
○ Urine
○ sugar
○ WR
○ Lipid profile?
○ e.c.g.?
○ Chest X-ray?
○ Skull X-ray?

Consider

○ aids to adapt the home ⎫
○ meals on wheels   ⎬ social worker
○ home help   ⎪
○ aids for rehabilitation ⎪
○ financial assistance   ⎭

○ home nursing services   – district
                              nurse
○ primary care team support – GP
                            – HV
                            – practice
                              nurse

○ attendance at local day ⎫
   centre, day hospital or ⎪
   rehabilitation unit   ⎬ hospital
○ occupational therapy   ⎪ resources
○ physiotherapy   ⎪
○ speech therapy   ⎭
   (of little value)
○ stroke clubs

NOTE:
A. Depression is a common complication of stroke
B. Aspirin antiplatelet activity may help stop TIAs going onto full stroke
C. Support family as well as patient

E5 Gastrointestinal

Dyspepsia and Functional Disorders of the GI Tract

What are they

A mixed bag of symptoms of disordered function relating to the GI tract. They include from above downwards – heartburn, flatulence, nausea, upper abdominal discomfort, mid and lower pains, constipation and loose frequent stools.
Although classified together their causes, nature, course and outcome are far from clear.

Possible causes

Organic (to be excluded)
○ hiatus hernia
○ peptic ulcer
○ neoplasms
○ GB and liver disease
○ Crohn's disease
○ diverticulosis
○ post-infective

Non-organic (to be considered)
○ emotion of pyschosomatic and stress factors
○ diet – such as lack of roughage, or too much roughage, and sensitivities to sugar, milk, coffee, tea, tobacco, etc.
○ iatrogenic factors – such as laxatives, aspirin, codeine, etc.
○ family history

Significance

Frequency – annual prevalence
○ heartburn, flatulence, nausea and upper abdo. discomfort – 21 per 1000 (55 patients per GP)
○ abdominal pains – 15 per 1000 (45 per GP)
○ constipation – diarrhoea – 8 per 1000 (20 per GP)
○ sex distribution – roughly equal

Assessments

○ first steps are to consider possibility of non-organic disorder
○ second step must be to exclude possible organic disorders and series of investigations are necessary
○ third step must be to avoid going on and on with more and more investigations.

Planned care

Bear in mind that –
○ disorders are common
○ since causes are unclear there can be no effective specific treatment
○ they are benign with a tendency to remit spontaneously and naturally.

Therefore no satisfactory planned care is possible.

Each GP should develop his own understanding of these patients and of possible advice and medication.

Peptic Ulcers

What are they

Symptom-complexes plus evidence of duodenal or gastric ulceration. Ulceration may be demonstrated by
○ radiography
○ endoscopy
○ at surgery
○ at autopsy

Significance

○ incidence – 3 per 1000 per year (7–8 new cases per GP)
○ prevalence – 15 per 1000 per year (35–40 patients per GP)
○ duodenal:gastric ulcers = 4 > 1
○ sex distribution – DU – M > F = 3 : 1
                          GU – M > F = 1 : 1

Natural history

Duodenal ulcers
○ onset usually at 20–40 years
○ recurrent bouts of symptoms for 5–10 years
○ 70% tend to remit naturally and cease to suffer symptoms
○ 30% will become chronic or develop complications and may require surgery

Gastric ulcers
○ onset usually at 40–60
○ 75% tend to heal spontaneously
○ 25% may need surgery

Assessment

Diagnostic features
○ central epigastric pain related to meals and relieved by food and antacids
○ vomiting – if pyloric spasm or obstruction
○ reflux and heart – if hiatus hernia or lax gastro-oesophageal sphincter
○ periodic bouts of pain

Complication
○ bleeding
         ○ haematemesis
         ○ melaena
○ perforation
○ malignant change in GU
○ stenosis of pylorus

Investigations

Confirm by
○ barium meal radiography
○ endoscopy (if indicated)

Differentiate from
○ 'non-ulcer dyspepsia'
○ hiatus hernia
○ gall bladder disease˙
○ pancreatic cancer
○ large gut cancers

Associated diseases
Note special tendency for DU patients to suffer from
○ IHD
○ chronic bronchitis
○ pulmonary TB
○ anxiety – depression

Planned care

Patient
○ understand nature and course of condition
○ trigger and aggravating factors
○ diet control (by trial and error)
○ relief measures (medication)

GP
○ understand natural history
○ confirm diagnosis (by Ba. Meal)
○ therapeutic plans
○ consider referral

Specialist
○ physician or surgeon?
○ to confirm diagnosis by endoscopy
○ to advise on therapy (in problem cases)
○ to carry out surgery

Principles of management

○ inform patient of diagnosis, nature and course of disorder
○ advise on lifestyle and habits
○ advise on trigger factors
○ diet
    ○ be as simple, clear and flexible as possible
    ○ avoid foods known to upset
    ○ frequent small meals

○ antacids
    ○ very effective in controlling pain temporarily

○ antispasmodics
    ○ no good evidence that they work
    ○ carbenoxolone and deglychirrhizinzed liquorice shown to work
      well in gastric ulcers
    ○ note side effects – fluid retention

○ histamine (H_2) - antagonists (cimetidine and ranitidine)

    major advance and effective in reducing acid production
    ○ expensive – apparently few side effects
    ○ use with sense and sensibility

○ surgery
    ○ very effective in selected cases
    ○ vagotomy now in fashion
    ○ partial gastrectomy in some
    ○ surgical mortality now 0.1–1% (depends on unit)
    ○ decline in rate of surgery since introduction of H_2-antagonists

Irritable Bowel Syndrome (spastic colon, mucous colitis)

What is it

A stress disorder in a susceptible individual with small and large bowel excessive motility associated with abdominal pain ranging from slight discomfort to severe colic, constipation or diarrhoea.

Aetiology

Appears to be closely related to emotional conflict and associated with depression. Marital conflict, bereavement, obsessional worry over often trivial matters.

Significance

○ symptoms may be similar in early ulcerative colitis, diverticulosis, intestinal malignancy or infection. May be presenting symptoms of a functional disorder such as depression and/or anxiety
○ failure to diagnose correctly may lead to severe iatrogenic reactions

Assessment

○ diagnosed by very careful study of history and response to treatment with anxiolytics and anticholinergics plus patient listening by doctor
○ radiological investigation such as *Barium enema* indicated at least once to reassure patient (and doctor)
○ bear in mind paucity of symptoms and signs of early colonic malignancy
○ sigmoidoscopy necessary to exclude ulcerative colitis or neoplasms

Clinical types

○ spastic type with variable bowel movements (constipation or diarrhoea) and colonic type pain in one or more areas. Relieved by bowel movement and often 'triggered off' by meal. Associated with depression, anxiety and fatigue
○ painless loose stools. Urgent diarrhoea after meals or on rising

Planned care

○ explain 'cause and effect' to patient
○ advise normal diet. Encourage bulk cereal such as muesli base, bran and wheat germ
○ may be necessary to give anticholinergic agents such as propanthleline with or without a tranquillizer such as diazepam
○ may have to treat with an antidepressant such as amitriptyline
○ sympathy and understanding from doctor most important

Gallbladder Disease

What is it

Chronic or acute inflammation of the mucosal lining often associated with the presence of stones.

Many theories as to cause. Insoluble cholesterol made soluble in gallbladder by mixing with bile acids and phospholipids.

Precipitation leads to stone formation which in turn may, by mechanical obstruction and trauma to mucosa, facilitate infection thus sustaining chain of pathological changes within the organ.

Significance

○ incidence – 0.5% per 1000 (1 new patient per year per GP)
○ prevalence – 2 per 1000 (5 patients per GP)
○ more common in females. May mimic disease of cardiac origin, e.g. angina or infarction, may present like peptic ulcer or appendicitis

Assessment

○ history important
○ flatulent dyspepsia
○ pain and tenderness
○ R. upper quadrant
○ positive Murphy's sign
○ straight X-ray and cholecystogram

Clinical types

Gallstones	Acute cholecystitis	Chronic cholecystitis
60% asymptomatic	pain night or early a.m.	very ill defined
upper abdominal discomfort	localized tenderness	flatulence may be only symptom
belching and food intake	nausea & vomit fever	pain usually **not** colicky

Treatment

○ many patients live asymptomatically with gallstones and gallbladders
○ surgical referral if symptoms persist or complications such as jaundice and if diagnosis is uncertain

E6 Endocrine

Diabetes Mellitus

What is it

A diabetic has a persistent abnormally high blood glucose concentration. Such a person will usually have glycosuria but not everyone with glycosuria has diabetes nor does every diabetic have glycosuria at all times because of varying thresholds.

Significance

○ incidence – 1.5 per 1000 (3–4 new patients per GP in year)
○ prevalence – 7 per 1000 (15–20 patients per GP)

Main types of diabetes and presenting features

	Insulin dependent (Juvenile onset)	Non-insulin dependent (Maturity onset)
Thirst and polyuria	Usual	Unusual
Loss of weight	Usual	Unusual
Obesity	Uncommon	Frequent
Ketosis	Usual	Unusual
Onset	Acute	Gradual
Incidence	<40 years (peak 12–14 years) Seasonal (peak during winter)	>40 years (rises with age)
Genetic predisposition	Strong: linked to HLA type	Present: not linked to HLA type

Assessment

Insulin dependent: In the young, the condition usually presents as an emergency with thirst, polyuria, loss of weight and ketosis with pallor, sweating, air hunger and smell of acetone.

Non-insulin dependent: May present with complications such as leg ulcers or retinopathy or be found by routine urine or blood test.

Blood glucose concentrations

	Fasting	Random	2 hours after 50 g glucose by mouth (e.g. 235 ml Lucozade)
Normal	<90 mg/100 ml (5.0 mmol/l)	<160 mg/100 ml (8.9 mmol/l)	<110 mg/100 ml (6.1 mmol/l)
Diabetes	>120 mg/100 ml (6.7 mmol/l)	>180 mg/100 ml (10 mmol/l)	>180 mg/100 ml (10 mmol/l)

Concentrations between these levels may indicate impaired glucose tolerance and require an oral glucose tolerance test (G.T.T.)

Complications

The exact mechanism is not clear but all seem to be related to hyper-glycaemia and so strict control is worth striving for.

Organ	Pathology	Effect	Management
Eyes	Retinopathy	Loss of vision	Improve control + photo-coagulation in suitable cases.
	Cataract	Loss of vision	Improve control + surgery in suitable cases
	Ocular nerve palsies	Diplopia	Improve control
Kidneys	Glomerular disease	Proteinuria Nephrotic syndrome	Improve control Low protein diet if uraemic
		Hypertension	Antihypertensives necessary
	Arterial disease	Renal failure Hypertension Renal failure	
	Pyelonephritis	Loss of diabetic control	Improve control
		Fever, pain, malaise	Antibiotics
CVS	**Generalized atheroma of both small and large arteries**		Improve control. Stop smoking. Reduce dietary animal fats
	Ischaemic heart disease	Angina, cardiac infarction	As in non-diabetic
	Cerebrovascular disease	C.V.A., dementia	
	Peripheral vascular disease	Intermittent claudication	Foot care
		Peripheral gangrene	Amputation may be necessary
CNS	**Neuropathies**		
	Sensory	Paraesthesiae Trophic ulcers	Improve control
	Motor	Peripheral nerve palsies	
	Autonomic	Impotence GI disturbance	
Skin	Infection		
	○ bacterial ○ fungal	Foot sepsis Ulcers	Improve control Foot care. Chiropody
	Ischaemia	Peripheral gangrene	Local treatment of infection
	Trophic ulcers		
	Necrobiosis		

Planned care

Aims:
○ to maintain blood sugar as near normal as possible
○ to prevent, delay and ameliorate complications
○ to enable the patient to live as normal a life as possible

Initial stabilization

Insulin dependent	Non-insulin dependent
In hospital Acute illness controlled by frequent doses of short acting insulin preparation and treatment of electrolyte imbalance	**At home** Target weight agreed Diet laid down
Basic dosage regimen established Injection technique taught Experience of hypoglycaemia arranged	Oral hypoglycaemic agents needed only if diet alone inadequate. Unlikely to be needed if patient overweight and dieting. May become necessary once target weight has been reached
Principles of diet explained Urine (or blood) testing taught	Urine testing taught

Insulin
○ always needed by anyone who has ever had ketosis
○ insulin is available in its original form (obtained from either beef or pig) or in highly purified (monocomponent) form; also in preparations of varying length of action.

	Original (standard)	Highly purified (Monocomponent)
Short acting	Soluble insulin	Neutral insulin, e.g. Actrapid MC
Intermediate length of action	Globin zinc insulin	Isophane insulin (NPH) e.g. Insulin Leo Retard Zinc suspension semilente e.g. Semitard MC
Long acting	Protamine zince insulin (PZI)	Zinc suspension ultralente e.g. Ultratard MC
Fixed mixtures of the above	Zinc suspension lente	Biphasic insulin, e.g. Rapitard MC Zinc suspension lente e.g. Monotard MC

The best control is usually obtained with twice daily injections: before breakfast and before the evening meal. These should each contain a short acting preparation. In addition, the morning injection may have a long acting insulin or an intermediate acting preparation may be added to either or both. The exact relative dosage can only be worked out after the patient has left hospital, has reached his target weight and is leading a normal life.

More accurate control can be achieved by combinations of preparations mixed by the patient than by using standard preparations of mixtures. The patient can then alter the dose to allow for times of varying activity such as sport or lazy weekends.

Types and strengths of insulin, with a guide to onset and length of action.

Preparation		Manufacturer	Strength i,u/ml						Onset, peak activity and duration of action in hours (approx.)
			20	40	80	100	320		
Insulin Injection	*Soluble*	Boots / CP Pharm. / Wellcome	● / ●	● / ● / ●	● / ● / ●	●	●	
Neutral Insulin Injection	*Neutral*	Evans				●		
	Actrapid MC	Novo		●	●	●		
	Human Actrapid (emp)	Novo		●	●	●		
	Human Velosulin (emp)	Nordisk and Wellcome				●		
	Humulin S (crb)	Lilly		●	●	●		
	Hypurin Neutral	CP Pharm.		●		●		
	Neusulin	Wellcome		●		●		
	Quicksol	Boots		●	●	●		
	Velosulin	Nordisk and Wellcome		●	●	●		
Biphasic Insulin Injection	Human Initard 50/50 (emp)	Nordisk and Wellcome				●		
	Human Mixtard 30/70 (emp)	Nordisk and Wellcome				●		
	Initard 50/50	Nordisk and Wellcome		●	●	●		
	Mixtard 30/70	Nordisk and Wellcome		●	●	●		
	Rapitard MC	Novo		●	●	●		
Insulin Zinc Suspension (Amorphous)	*Semilente*	Boots Wellcome		●	●			
	Semitard MC	Novo		●	●	●		
Isophane Insulin Injection	*Isophane (NPH)*	Boots Evans		●	●	●		
	Human Insulatard (emp)	Nordisk and Wellcome				●		
	Human Protaphane (emp)	Novo				●		
	Humulin I (crb)	Lilly		●	●	●		
	Hypurin Isophane	CP Pharm.		●	●	●		
	Insulatard	Nordisk and Wellcome		●	●	●		
	Monophane	Boots				●		
	Neuphane	Wellcome		●	●	●		
Insulin Zinc Suspension (Mixed)	*Lente*	Boots Evans			●	●		
	Human Monotard (emp)	Novo		●	●	●		
	Hypurin Lente	CP Pharm.				●		
	Lentard MC	Novo		●	●	●		
	Monotard MC	Novo		●	●	●		
	Neulente	Wellcome		●	●	●		
	Tempulin	Boots				●		
Insulin Zinc Suspension (Crystalline)	*Ultralente*	Boots Wellcome			●			
	Human Ultratard (emp)	Novo				●		
	Humulin Zn (crb)	Lilly				●		
	Ultratard MC	Novo		●	●	●		
Protamine Zinc Insulin Injection	*Protamine Zinc*	Boots Wellcome		●	●			
	Hypurin Protamine Zinc	CP Pharm.			●	●		

Oral hypoglycaemic agents
O should not be used until target weight has been reached and treatment
  with diet alone has been continued for at least 3 weeks
O should be used in conjunction with diet.
O not suitable for anyone who has ever had ketosis
O interactions with other drugs are common.

	Action	Advantages	Disadvantages
Sulphonyl ureas	Mainly by stimulating insulin release	Well tolerated	Increase in weight. Risk of hypoglycaemia
Biguanides	Mixture of actions including delay of glucose absorption from bowel	Decrease in weight	Gastrointestinal disturbance. Risk of lactic acidosis

Group	Name	Daily dose	Characteristics
Sulphonyl ureas	Tolbutamide	1–3 g	Shortest acting: least potent: least likely to cause hypoglycaemia: suitable for elderly
	Chlorpropamide	100–375mg	Long acting (24 hours or more): more potent: may cause hypoglycaemia: may cause flushing with alcohol: mildly antidiuretic
	Glibenclamide	2.5–25mg	As potent as chlorpropamide: shorter acting than chlorpropamide: mildly diuretic
Biguanides	Phenformin	50–150mg	Especially useful in obese patient or in conjunction with sulphonyl-ureas
	Metformin	0.5–2 g	

Education: continues throughout the life of the patient

For all diabetics:	Principles of diet: ○ no sugar ○ restriction of other carbohydrates and animal fats ○ regular meals of equal calorie content evenly spaced ○ no binges
	Importance of weight control
	Urine testing for glucose with Clinitest tablets if renal threshold normal (Clinistix or Diastix can be used but less accurate).
	Several tests during an occasional typical day at different times are more use than one every day at the same time
	Blood testing with Dextostix and meter allows more accurate control than urine testing. Essential if renal threshold abnormal. Useful in pregnancy
	Importance of accurate control and follow-up
	Recognition of danger signs, e.g. vomiting
	Foot care
	No smoking
For insulin dependent:	Siting and technique of injections
	Adjustment of dosage according to tests and needs
	Factors affecting insulin requirement, e.g. illness and reduced exercise increase requirement: increased exercise and reduced calorie intake reduce requirement
	Types of insulin being used and their length of action
	Symptoms of hypoglycaemia: sweating, shakiness, pallor, forceful heart beat, fearfulness, irritability, acute intense hunger, nightmares, poor concentration
	Factors likely to cause hypoglycaemia, e.g. increased exertion, missed meals, increased insulin dosage (or wrong strength)
	Management of hypoglycaemic attacks: ○ emergency – sugar ○ long term – reduce insulin
	NOTE: The emergency use of sugar for the treatment of hypoglycaemia may cause glycosuria and lead the patient to think he needs more insulin and not less
	Maintenance of target weight: ○ if underweight – increase dietary intake especially of protein foods, fruit and vegetables; increase dose of insulin as necessary, adjudged by tests ○ if overweight – reduce calorie intake and dose of insulin. When target weight is reached, insulin dose will need to be increased again
For non-insulin dependent:	Tablet taking routine
	Drug interaction

Planned long-term care	○ collaboration between GP, diabetes health visitor or hospital diabetic clinic, plus ophthalmologist. ○ intervals may need to be shorter in the unstable, unintelligent or those with complications.

Every 6 months
○ education
○ check patient's chart for urine (or blood) tests
○ enquire for hypoglycaemic symptoms
○ review diet
○ record weight
○ examine feet in middle-aged and elderly
○ test urine for albumin
○ take blood for random blood sugar or HbA₁C.

Note: HbA₁C (glycosylated haemoglobin)
○ Percentage of HbA glycosylated is directly proportional to the time the red cell has been exposed to glucose and the height of the glucose levels. It therefore provides a useful assessment of mean blood glucose control over several weeks.
○ Result of 10–20% signifies uncontrolled diabetes; < 8% is normal or good control (**NB** occasionally may reflect frequent and dangerous episodes of hypoglycaemia).
○ Once or twice yearly measurements provide a very useful guide to overall control.

Once a year
○ eye check (by ophthalmologist)
○ check peripheral circulation
○ blood pressure
○ examine injection sites
○ examine tendon reflexes and deep pain sensation
○ MSU and dip inoculum (early morning).

Self-help

○ probably more important than for any other condition
○ self-responsibilities for diet, medication and control
○ information from:
> British Diabetic Association,
> 10 Queen Anne Street,
> London W1M 0BD.

Guidelines	○ make sure of diagnosis

Guidelines
- ○ make sure of diagnosis
- ○ decide on type of diabetes
- ○ assess general health and advice on
  - ○ non-smoking
  - ○ regular normal living
  - ○ weight control
  - ○ exercise

- ○ **insulin**
  - ○ required only in about one quarter of diabetics
  - ○ absolute or relative indications
    - ○ pre-coma, coma
    - ○ ketosis
    - ○ children – juveniles
    - ○ under weight
    - ○ complications

- ○ **diet and weight control**
  - ○ for all diabetics

- ○ **oral hypoglycaemics**
  - ○ only after a trial of diet and weight control
  - ○ supplement diet and not replace it

Organization of care

Wherever the care is to be provided and whoever is to be responsible, a clear planned programme of care has to be agreed and adhered to.

Diabetic diet

Diabetics are provided with diet sheets from a number of different sources including those from hospital dietitians and the British Diabetic Association.

Unfortunately none of these seem to take account of modern medical ideas on what diabetics should eat. It may be better to provide a set of guidelines which may be used alone or to modify existing diets.

Quantity
Eat as much as you need to keep fit and well and active.

Eat at regular intervals throughout the day.

If you are underweight, eat more or increase your insulin or both.

If you are overweight, eat less or decrease your insulin, or both.

Content
Eat **plenty** of the following:
Fruit of all kinds including bananas
Vegetables of all kinds, including potatoes, beans, peas and rice
Wholemeal bread
Cereals (not sugary ones)
Fish – cooked without fat

Eat **moderate amounts** of the following:
Lean meat
Skimmed milk
Margarine high in polyunsaturated fats
Cottage cheese

Eat **very little** of the following:
    Eggs: maximum three per week including those in cooking
    Whole milk cheeses, e.g cheddar
    Foods containing sugar and/or fats, e.g. biscuits, cake
    Salt

Eat **none** of these:
    Fat meat; sausages, bacon, beefburgers, pork in any form
    Cream cheeses
    Cream
    Butter
    Whole milk
    Sugar
    Fruit squashes, jams, sweets, chocolates, ice cream

Thyroid

HYPOTHALAMUS

TRH: (thyrotrophin-releasing hormone) secreted by hypothalamus stimulates ant. pituitary to produce TSH.

ANT. PITUITARY

Thyroid hormones:
T_3 (triiodothyronine) and T_4 (tetraiodothyronine or thyroxine) inhibit production of TSH by ant. pituitary.

TSH: (thyroid stimulating hormone) secreted by ant. pituitary stimulates thyroid to produce thyroid hormones T_3 and T_4.

THYROID

The feedback mechanism: the thyroid gland produces two main hormones: thyroxine (tetraiodothyronine or T_4) and T_3 (triiodothyronine). In the normal state, the production of these and their release into the circulation is under the control of the anterior pituitary by means of thyroid stimulating hormone (TSH) which in turn is controlled by thyrotrophin-releasing hormone (TRH) from the hypothalamus. When the circulating levels of T_3 and T_4 rise the anterior pituitary produces less TSH and the thyroid gland becomes less active, producing and releasing less T_3 and T_4.

Most of the thyroid hormones in the circulation are bound to proteins. It is only the free (unbound) hormones which are metabolically active.

Hyperthyroidism

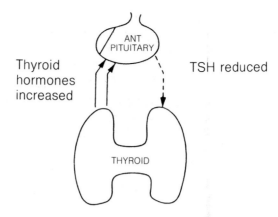

In hyperthyroidism, the thyroid gland is autonomous and no longer under the control of TSH. The level of the circulating free thyroid hormones (T_3 and T_4) is increased and the anterior pituitary therefore produces little or no TSH.

Hypothyroidism

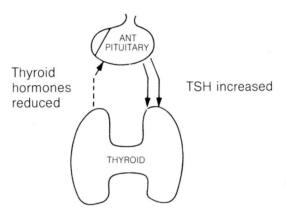

In hypothyroidism, the thyroid gland fails to respond to TSH. The circulating level of free thyroid hormones is reduced and that of TSH increased.

Diseases of the
thyroid gland

Goitre	Hyperthyroidism	Hypothyroidism
Physiological in puberty and pregnancy **In hyperthyroidism** e.g. Graves' disease (an autoimmune disease) Toxic nodular goitre. **In hypothyroidism** e.g. iodine deficiency **Benign** – adenomata and cysts **Carcinoma**	Abnormally high circulating free thyroid hormones (mostly T_3) Goitre may or may not be present	Abnormally low circulating free thyroid hormones Goitre may or may not be present **Primary:** ○ iodine deficiency ○ agenesis of thyroid gland ○ antithyroid drugs ○ autoimmune thyroiditis (e.g. Hashimoto's) ○ following ^{131}iodine treatment ○ following surgery **Secondary:** ○ to pituitary disease (rare) ○ to hypothalamic disease (very rare)

Significance –
what happens?

Hyperthyroidism	Hypothyroidism
Increase in oxygen consumption, basal metabolic rate and metabolism of carbohydrates, proteins and fats. Increased activity of sympathetic nervous system accounts for many of the symptoms and signs. Untreated, the increase in cardiac output and hyperpyrexia cause the main problems.	**Neonatal** – ○ prolonged jaundice ○ large tongue with noisy breathing and feeding difficulties ○ lethargy **In children** – failure of growth, development and maturation (Cretinism) **In adults** – general retardation of all systems, depositing of mucoid substance in skin, tongue and vocal cords

	Hyperthyroidism	Hypothyroidism
Commonest symptoms	Feeling warm – intolerance of heat	Lethargy
		Feeling cold
	Loss of weight, increased appetite, diarrhoea	Weight gain
		Loss of hair
	Palpitations, shortness of breath (especially important in the elderly)	Dryness of skin
		Hoarseness of voice
	Increased fatigueability	Amenorrhoea (especially in young)
	Feeling fidgety	Menorrhagia (especially in aged)
	Irritability, nervousness	Constipation
		Puffy eyelids
Most important physical signs	Warm skin, sweating	Movement and thought slow
	Evidence of loss of weight	Voice hoarse and speech slow
	Tachycardia	Skin coarse and thickened, sallow
	Systolic hypertension with high pulse pressure	Hair dry and brittle
	Systolic murmur	Periphery cyanosed and cold
	Fine tremor	Relaxation of tendon jerks delayed
	Exophthalmos, lid retraction (appearance of sclera between upper lid and limbus of cornea when patient is looking straight ahead) In the elderly, signs of heart failure of atrial fibrillation be the only findings.	Less common: psychosis (myxoedema madness), coma, carpal tunnel syndrome, deafness, aches and pains, cardiac ischaemia, anaemia, hypothermia
	Goitre: may be difficult to detect or retrosternal – presence of thyroid bruit helpful	

Assessment – diagnosis

The diagnosis is made on clinical grounds, but tests may help.

| Tests of thyroid function | ### Serum T4 concentration
Raised in hyperthyroidism, lowered in hypothyroidism. Simple, cheap, and reliable but is a measure of the total circulating thyroxine and not just of the free thyroxine. It depends on the concentration of binding proteins especially thyroxine-binding globulin (TBG). The level of serum TBG may be affected by a number of different conditions, and especially by drugs, making the serum T4 concentrations alone an inaccurate measure of thyroid function. Some drugs occupy TBG binding sites normally available to thyroxine reducing the total serum T4 concentration.

Free thyroxine index
This may be useful if an alteration of TBG is suspected of influencing the serum T4 concentration. It is calculated from the serum T4 and the residual binding capacity of the TBG (i.e. the amount of TBG not bound to thyroxine) expressed in terms of 'serum T3 uptake' or 'resin uptake'. The significance of the result depends on the type of test used. It is important to check with the laboratory the expected direction of change in each condition.

Serum TBG
Can be measured but test not yet generally available. May replace T3 uptake tests in future.

Serum TSH
Very low or undetectable in normal people and in hyperthyroidism; high or very high in hypothyroidism. Reverts to normal with treatment.

Serum T3
More difficult and expensive than Serum T4. High in hyperthyroidism when T4 also raised. Raised in T3 toxicosis when T4 normal (rare).

Summary
Hyperthyroidism: Serum T4 increased (usually)
Hypothyroidism: Serum T4 reduced (usually)
                  TSH raised (always)
○ important to state clinical details on pathology request form.
○ if diagnosis uncertain, wait a few months and re-assess.
○ hyperthyroidism may become more obvious during hot weather.
○ cancer should always be suspected in non-toxic nodular goitre. |

| Planned care | ### Hyperthyroidism:
May be undertaken entirely by general practitioner except for surgery and radioactive iodine for which appropriate referrals are required.

Immediate:
If severely affected:
○ rest
○ β-blocker: e.g. propanolol 40 mg b.d. increasing to 160 mg b.d. if necessary within a few days to control tachycardia, tremor, sweating, etc.
NOTE: check no symptoms or signs of heart failure or history of asthma.
○ carbimazole: check WBC before starting. 10 mg t.d.s. until euthyroid (4–6 weeks). Warn patient to report any sore throat immediately.
○ in mild cases rest and β-blocker may not be needed. |

Planned care
continued

Medium-term
When patient euthyroid:
○ tail off β-blocker
○ reduce carbimazole to 5–15 mg daily (monitor dose on basis of clinical signs, not on blood tests).
○ check WBC every 2 weeks for first 2 months.
○ decide on longer term management:
　　○ antithyroid drugs
　　○ surgery
　　○ radioactive iodine.

Long term:
Antithyroid drugs: (carbimazole or propylthiouracil).
○ agranulocytosis is a rare toxic effect occurring only during the first 2 months. Sensitivity may occur in the form of rashes, arthralgia, jaundice.
○ treatment is continued for 12–18 months.
○ relapse is common and the patient should be reviewed regularly after cessation of treatment.

Surgery (partial thyroidectomy)
○ treatment of choice if goitre large, causing pressure symptoms or the patient is sensitive to or unwilling to take carbimazole.
○ patient should be euthyroid before operation.
○ hyperthyroidism may recur or hypothyroidism develop so long term follow up is necessary.

Radioactive iodine (^{131}I)
○ treatment of choice for most patients over 45 years. Previously held fears of cancer or leukaemia appear to be unfounded. May be 6–10 weeks before fully effective. Second or third dose may be needed but not less than 4 months between.
○ many patients eventually become hypothyroid.
○ all should be reviewed by general practitioner at intervals for 20 years (every 3 months for 1 year, every 5 months for next 2 years, then annually).

Thyrotoxicosis in pregnancy:
○ treat as in the non-pregnant patient but radioactive iodine cannot be used.

Hypothyroidism:
Ambulant treatment by general practitioner usually best unless the patient is in heart failure or coma when hospital referral may be necessary.

L-Thyroxine sodium (Eltroxin) tablets: 100–200 μg once a day. The dose should be monitored on the basis of the clinical response.
Thyroid function tests cannot be used for this purpose. The serum TSH falls to normal when the condition is treated but no further falls may be detected if the dose of thyroxine is too high.

In the elderly or anyone with angina or heart failure, treatment must be started with a very low dose, e.g. 50 μg daily and increased gradually every 2–3 weeks.

General:
○ practice register of all diagnosed thyroid patients (hypo- and hyper-).
○ arrange at least one annual assessment (clinical and perhaps tests) for rest of their lives.

E7   Genitourinary

Chronic Renal Failure

What is it

○ slow and progressive decline in renal function with uraemic syndrome and death as end points.
○ should be reversible with modern therapies.

○ **causes**
    ○ chronic glomerulonephritis (primary and secondary)
    ○ chronic pyelonephritis
    ○ diabetic nephropathy
    ○ drug nephropathy
    ○ chronic urinary tract outflow obstruction
    ○ high blood pressure
    ○ gout
    ○ polycystic kidneys
    ○ myeloma
    ○ amyloid

Significance

○ prognosis depends on causes and whether they are correctable.
○ reversible with dialysis and/or transplantation.
○ early diagnosis and referral to specialist nephrology unit are best.
○ care is long term, expensive, time consuming and requiring much self-help and collaboration.
○ outlook good with long term dialysis (75%: 2-year survival) and renal transplantation (50%: 2-year survival).

Assessment

○ clinical for primary disease and of individual patient and family.
○ full blood check for anaemia.
○ blood urea and creatinine clearance for renal function.
○ serum uric acid for gout.
○ urography and tomography – for renal size and obstruction
○ midstream urine for infection.
○ serum calcium, phosphate and alkaline phosphatase for renal bone disease.

Principles of management and planned care

○ **personal patient and family care and support** of great importance by hospital, GP and community services working in liaison.

○ **preservation of remaining nephrons**
    ○ control high blood pressure and heart failure.
    ○ control urinary infection
    ○ correct urinary tract obstructions.
    ○ maintain water–salt balance.
    ○ care with drug use.

○ **conservative management of uraemia**
    ○ low protein diet.
    ○ aluminium hydroxide to delay renal bone disease.
    ○ vitamin D and calcium to correct low calcium levels.
    ○ allopurinol to control raised serum uric acid.

○ **long term dialysis** – indications:
    ○ 5–55-year-olds without systemic disease.
    ○ progressive deterioration of renal function.
    ○ complications such as renal bone disease and pericarditis.

○ **renal transplant**
    ○ consider for all on long term dialysis with no chronic infection or bladder flow obstruction.

Urinary Tract Infection

What is it

○ **Acute cystitis**
  - Infection confined to the bladder
  - Impossible to demonstrate bacteriuria in about 50%. Uncertain whether this is due to absence of true infection or technological inadequacy
  - Recurrent attacks of frequency and dysuria without demonstrable bacteriuria known as urethral syndrome

○ **Acute pyelitis**
  - Infection of renal pelvis and ureter

Significance
  - May be associated with congenital abnormality, especially in children
  - Important in pregnancy
  - May indicate sexual problem

Assessment
  - Diagnosis can be made with certainty only by MSU, preferably EMU with dip innoculin
  - In children:
    ○ important to be certain of diagnosis even if this means delaying treatment
    ○ further investigation required after one confirmed attack in a boy, after two in a girl
  - MSU not necessary in isolated attack of acute cystitis in an otherwise healthy young woman

	Acute cystitis	Acute pyelitis
Symptoms	Mainly local: frequency, dysuria, haematuria, lower abdominal pain	Mainly general: fever, rigours abdominal pain, headache, vomiting, failure to thrive in infants
	Some general: nausea, malaise, fever	Some local: frequency, loin pain
Incidence	Common in sexually active women and anyone with abnormal urinary tract	In **Infants**: more common in boys than girls
	Common in elderly women	In **adults**: more common in women especially in pregnancy
		Often associated with abnormal urinary tract
Pathogenesis	Bacterial infection ascending from vulva via urethra. >75% *E. coli*	Sometimes ascending, i.e. secondary to cystitis
		Sometimes haematogenous (especially in infants)
Predisposing factors	Poor hygiene resulting in high population of pathogens around urethral meatus	Congenital abnormality
		Obstruction to lower urinary tract.
		Vesico-ureteric reflux
	Poor sexual technique causing trauma to urethral meatus	Renal damage, e.g. scars, analgesic nephropathy, ischaemia
	Infrequent voiding	Bacteriuria during pregnancy
	Residual urine, e.g. associated with bladder neck obstruction, vesico-ureteric reflux, foreign bodies or diverticula	Calculi Neoplasms

Planned Care	○ **Acute cystitis** Single acute attack:

- 50% resolve within a few days with rest and increased fluid intake
Severe or persistent attacks:
- may be treated with antibiotics, e.g. trimethoprim 200 mg b.d. (avoid if risk of pregnancy) or amoxicillin 250 mg t.d.s. for 3 days. The last dose should be taken at bedtime whichever antibiotic is used
- fluid intake should be reduced to normal levels while antibiotics are being taken

Recurrent acute attacks:
- MSU to identify organism and sensitivies
- usually respond to intensive course of antibiotic as above followed by small prophylactic dose, e.g. trimethoprim 100 mg nocte or nitrofurantoin 100 mg nocte for a few weeks, or months, or after intercourse
- may require further investigations (see under pyelitis)
- advice on local hygiene and sexual technique may be useful

○ **Acute pyelitis**
Immediate
- MSU and dip inoculin
- Start antibiotic, e.g. amoxicillin 500 mg t.d.s. without waiting for result
- Bed rest
- Repeat MSU after 5–7 days before end of course of antibiotic

Later
- repeat MSU and dip inoculin after 2 weeks, 1 month and 3 months
- IVP
- Micturating cystourethrogram if residual urine found on IVP

Refer
- children
- anyone with structural abnormality
- anyone with recurrent attacks

Long term
- check BP and MSU at intervals and blood urea occasionally

E8   The Menopause

What is it

○ The end of menstruation; literally the last menstrual period.
○ Usually taken to include a variable time before and after during which problems may arise from both declining oestrogen production and social and domestic pressures.

Significance

○ Can be the source of much anxiety and unhappiness.
○ Can be associated with marital difficulty and problems with family relationships.
○ GP is in a position to make matters worse or to alleviate some of the problems.

Clinical presentation

○ About one third of menopausal women have no symptoms or only minimal ones.
○ A further one third have moderate symptoms which they may wish to discuss but which may need no treatment.
○ The final one third have distressing symptoms. These are:
  – hot flushes
  – dry vagina
  – irritability
  – emotional lability
  – depression
  – anxiety
  – insomnia.
○ Only the hot flushes and the dry vagina are the direct result of reduced oestrogen production.
○ Insomnia is commonly due to nocturnal hot flushes.
○ The emotional symptoms are at least partly due to social pressures: A menopausal woman is likely to
  – be needed less and less by her children, who may be leaving home or going through awkward adolescent stage
  – have reached a boring stage in her marriage
  – have no career or training which would enable her to get a well paid job
  – be unable to get a job at all
  – be financially dependent on her husband
  – have few hobbies or outside interests, having spent her life being a wife and mother
  – blame herself for all the problems in the family.

What to do

○ Listen **with interest and concern**
○ Explain, inform, interpret symptoms.
○ Present options
  – do nothing; the symptoms are likely to be intermittent and variable and may improve spontaneously soon
  – take non-hormone medication, e.g. pyridoxine or efamol (NOT tranquillizers)
  – take hormone replacement therapy (HRT) – provided there are no contraindications.

○ Watch for intercurrent illness:
  – hypothyroidism
  – anaemia
  – endogenous depression
○ Encourage general fitness:
  – keep slim
  – take exercise
  – healthy diet.

Hormone replacement therapy

○ Contraindications
Absolute – carcinoma of breast, cervix, uterus, ovary
  – history of thromboembolic episode.
Relative – obesity
  – diabetes
  – hypertension
  – smoking
  – liver disease

○ Indications
  – To prevent postmenopausal osteoporosis
    (a) in a woman who has had a hysterectomy and bilateral oophorectomy for benign disease: start immediately postoperatively.
    (b) in a woman who has had a hysterectomy for benign condition, start at 50–55 years.
        Continue until aged 70 years.
  – To treat hot flushes and/or dry vagina. Use for 3–6 months and then stop and see if need continues.

○ Before prescribing
  – check for contraindications
  – examine breasts and encourage future breast self-examination
  – check blood pressure
  – do vaginal examination and cervical smear
  – make sure the woman wants the drug
  – warn her that she may have menstrual-type bleeding every fourth week.

○ Prescribing HRT
  – for a woman with a uterus, oestrogen should be prescribed on a cyclical basis with a progestogen added in the second half of the cycle.
  – for a woman without a uterus, this may still be best but unopposed oestrogen, e.g. ethinyloestradiol 10–20 μg daily is often used.

○ Follow-up
  – see after 3 months to check blood pressure and progress.
  – if treatment is continued, repeat blood pressure and vaginal examination annually.

What not to do

○ Do not prescribe tranquillizers or hypnotics. To do so
  – confirms the woman's idea that she is unable to cope
  – limits her ability to deal with any difficulties she may have
  – leads to addiction
  – may cause depression.

E9　Non-illness

What is it

In general practice much of what is seen has no confirmed 'illness' labels.

○ **symptoms**

Many patients come with symptoms and problems that can never be clearly defined with any confirmatory investigations.

Tiredness, exhaustion, headaches, indigestion, various aches and pains and other symptoms are very real to the patient but no abnormalities can be discovered by the doctor on physical examination or investigation.

○ **social pathologies**

Many of the patients' problems are related to personal, family, work or environmental matters. Personal and family upsets, unemployment, money problems, crime, drugs, alcohol and the like can bring the patient to seek comfort and help.

○ **normal abnormalities**

Over one-half of work in general practice is with minor self-limiting conditions. Although they may produce recognizable 'syndromes' such as colds, backaches, acute D and V, stings and bites, cuts and bruises, dysmenorrhoea, premenstrual tension, vaginal discharge, nasal catarrh – these in some degrees are inevitable and have to be accepted as 'normal' to everyday life.

Significance

It has to be accepted that general practice is first contact care and that the general practitioner is the doctor of first contact. It is part of his role to act as the screener and assessor of undifferentiated and undiagnosed packages that patients decide to bring. Within such packages there has to be much 'non-illness', but often this can only be decided by a trained professional.

Non-illness has to be accepted as a part of general practice.

Assessment

○ do the symptoms have any organic basis?
○ do the symptoms fit any recognizable syndromes?
○ why has the patient come?
○ what underlying fears and problems?
○ what type of person?
○ what past history?
○ what family background?

Principles of management

○ patient
  ○ must be educated and informed of the nature of the 'non-illness' and instructed in future self-care.

○ the GP
  ○ must understand the significance of 'non-illness' and the likely reasons why the patient consults. The various forms of 'non-illness' should be recognized.
  ○ fears and anxieties should be anticipated and taken seriously.
  ○ the patient should be allowed to tell his story.
  ○ examination may be necessary more to reassure than in expectation of abnormal findings.
  ○ investigations and/or referral to a specialist may be necessary parts of the reassurance process.
  ○ social pathologies may not be curable but there are often ways of relieving their ill-effects.

○ specialist
  ○ must realize that referrals may be for positive reasons with negative pathologies.
  ○ referral letter should state the nature of the 'non-illness', the reasons why the patient is being referred and the actions that the GP expects, and hopes, the specialist to take.

General

○ it is best to accept 'non-illness' as a part of normal practice.
○ it is best that the GP develops a philosophy and a methodology to deal with it.

Index